Ethical Issues in Youth Work

Second edition

Edited by Sarah Banks

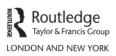
Routledge
Taylor & Francis Group

LONDON AND NEW YORK

First edition published 1999
by Routledge

This edition published 2010
by Routledge
2 Park Square, Milton Park, Abingdon, Oxon OX14 4RN

Simultaneously published in the USA and Canada
by Routledge
270 Madison Avenue, New York, NY 10016

Routledge is an imprint of the Taylor & Francis Group, an informa business

Typeset in Sabon
by Keystroke, Tettenhall, Wolverhampton
Printed and bound in Great Britain
by TJ International Ltd, Padstow, Cornwall

British Library Cataloguing in Publication Data
A catalogue record for this book is available from the British Library

Library of Congress Cataloging-in-Publication Data
Ethical issues in youth work / edited by Sarah Banks. — 2nd ed.
  p. cm.
Includes bibliographical references and index.
1. Youth workers—Professional ethics. 2. Social work with youth—Moral and
ethical aspects. I. Banks, Sarah.
[DNLM: 1. Social Work—ethics. 2. Adolescent. HV 1421 E84 2010]
HV1421.E74 2010
174′.93627—dc22   2009051664

ISBN10: 0–415–49970–4 (hbk)
ISBN10: 0–415–49971–2 (pbk)
ISBN10: 0–203–84936–1 (ebk)

ISBN13: 978–0–415–49970–5 (hbk)
ISBN13: 978–0–415–49971–2 (pbk)
ISBN13: 978–0–203–84936–1 (ebk)

Ethical Issues in Youth Work

This fully updated new edition of *Ethical Issues in Youth Work* presents a comprehensive overview and discussion of a range of ethical challenges facing youth workers in their everyday practice.

The first part offers a clear outline of the nature of professional ethics, relevant ethical theories and an overview of the policy and organisational context of youth work. The second part is grounded firmly in practice, with experts in the field exploring specific issues that raise ethical difficulties for youth workers, such as:

- when to breach confidentiality
- information sharing in inter-professional contexts
- the ethics of youth participation and active citizenship
- how to balance the roles of control, empowerment and education
- negotiating personal and professional values, interests and commitments in youth work
- dilemmas for faith-based and black and minority ethnic workers
- issues for practitioner researchers.

Ethical Issues in Youth Work offers a timely and unique insight into both the dilemmas of youth work practice and some of the more recent challenges faced by youth workers and all those working with young people in the light of current public attitudes and government policies towards young people.

Sarah Banks is Professor in the School of Applied Social Sciences at Durham University, UK.

Contents

Contributors

Sarah Banks is Professor in the School of Applied Social Sciences at Durham University, UK. She teaches and researches in the fields of youth, community and social work, with a particular interest in professional ethics. She is co-editor of the journal *Ethics and Social Welfare*, and co-director of the Centre for Social Justice and Community Action at Durham University.

Janet Batsleer works as Principal Lecturer in Youth and Community Work at Manchester Metropolitan University, where she has been based for the past 20 years or so. She is interested in the creativity of practice at all sorts of edges and margins, and remains actively involved in community-based projects in Manchester, particularly Forty Second Street and The Blue Room.

Rick Bowler is Senior Lecturer in Applied Community and Youth Work in the Faculty of Education and Society, University of Sunderland, where he is a member of the Centre for Equalities and Social Justice and the Centre for Children, Young People and Families. He is a past Chair of Young Asian Voices and of the Board of Directors of the North of England Refugee Service. He is currently working on a doctoral study into racisms and counter-racisms in and around youth work practice.

Maxine Green currently works as a consultant and specialises in faith-based youth work. Her interest in faith-based youth work was influenced by living as a Christian in a Muslim country for ten years and her work for the National Youth Office of the Church of England.

Umme F. Imam manages The Angelou Centre, an organisation promoting economic inclusion for black women in North East England. Previously she taught Community and Youth Work at Durham University. As a black woman, a strong commitment to highlighting the intersections of race and gender has underpinned her work as a practitioner and an academic.

Tony Jeffs teaches on youth and community work courses at Durham University and the University of Bedfordshire. He is a member of the Editorial Board of the journal *Youth and Policy*.

Kenneth McCulloch is a Senior Lecturer in Community Education at the University of Edinburgh. His interests are in young people and non-school, non-formal education, sail training, young people's citizenship and educational work to help young people become critical social actors.

Phil Mizen teaches sociology at the University of Warwick, UK. He has published extensively on youth and youth policy, with particular reference to young people, the labour market, welfare and the state. He is currently interested in the emergence of 'new urban childhoods' through research examining the survival strategies of children living under conditions of acute deprivation in Accra, Ghana.

Sue Morgan currently works for the National Trust at Shaw's Corner. She was a youth and community worker between 1980 and 2008, most recently based in secondary schools.

Howard Sercombe is Professor of Community Education at the University of Strathclyde, Glasgow. Originally from Australia, Howard has worked in a variety of settings, from inner-city detached work to community development in outback towns. He has a strong interest in youth work ethics, and has published widely on the subject.

Mark K. Smith is Rank Research Fellow and Tutor at the YMCA George Williams College, London.

Lyn Tett holds a personal Chair in Community Education and Lifelong Learning at the University of Edinburgh. Her interests lie within the broad area of community education and lifelong learning, and her research has involved an investigation of the factors such as class, gender and disability that lead to the exclusion of adults from post-compulsory education and of the action that might be taken to promote social inclusion.

Jason Wood is Head of Research in the Youth and Community Division at De Montfort University, Leicester. He recently completed a Ph.D. study that investigated how young people define and experience active citizenship; he has research and teaching interests in youth work, social policy and criminal justice. He co-edited *Work with Young People: Theory and Policy for Practice* (with Jean Hine, Sage) and is currently writing a book about young people and active citizenship.

Kerry Young has been involved in youth work since 1976, first as a part-time and later full-time detached youth worker. She has also worked for a number of national youth work organisations and is currently a youth work consultant and researcher at Harrington|Young organisation development consultants.

Preface and acknowledgements

I am delighted that it has been possible to compile a second edition of *Ethical Issues in Youth Work*. For a long time the first edition was the only book on the theme of ethics in youth work. It was published as part of a series on professional ethics for which the series editor was Ruth Chadwick. I am grateful to her for accepting the proposal for such a book in the 1990s when youth work was a relatively low-profile, small occupational group. Other books are now beginning to emerge on this topic. This is a good sign, as the late Jo Campling (my early mentor in the publishing field) always said – indicating a vibrant subject area and giving readers a choice of perspectives, styles and approaches. As an edited collection, this book covers a wide range of themes from a variety of perspectives – written by authors who are practitioners, managers, trainers and academics.

Naively, I thought that preparing a second edition would be a relatively easy task. However, the world has changed a lot since the late 1990s. Most chapters have been substantially revised, many completely rewritten and some new ones added. I am very grateful to the chapter authors for the enormous amount of work they have put into their chapters and for their patience with the endless rounds of revisions and amendments. I hope they feel the effort was worthwhile and that we have maintained the uniqueness of each author's voice, while adding standard features at the end of each chapter (questions for reflection and discussion and recommended reading). Rewriting a chapter after a decade is always a challenging task – causing uncomfortable reflections on the thoughts, arguments and modes of expression of the (former) self that wrote it, as well as requiring a laborious task of updating and reviewing changes in literature, policy and practice.

In addition to the chapter authors, I would like to thank Grace McInnes at Routledge for her positive support for this second edition and Khanam Virjee for keeping the project on track.

This book builds, of course, on the first edition, for which my colleague Tony Jeffs gave great encouragement. It also builds on the theorising and thinking of many authors, practitioners and students whose works have inspired us and with whom conversations have developed over the past decade. I owe a great debt to many people in the youth work field, who have contributed to keeping the profession alive and the debates moving, including: Filip Coussée, Aylssa Cowell, Bernard Davies, Chris Furze, Ruth Gilchrist, Don MacDonald, Anne Marron, Viv McKee, Bryan Merton, Leon Mexter, Doug Nicholls, John Rose, Alan Smith, Jean Spence, Tony Taylor, Howard Williamson and Tom Wylie. These are all people for whom the values and distinctiveness of youth work are important, worth fighting for and writing about. Hopefully this book is part of a broader project that is about developing and defending good youth work.

Introduction to the second edition

Sarah Banks

The first edition of *Ethical Issues in Youth Work* was published in 1999, with many chapters written during 1997 and 1998. Writing this introduction to the second edition in 2009 (anticipating the book's publication in 2010) provides an opportunity to reflect on the changes and developments in theory, policy and practice during the extended decade from 1997 to 2010.

Ethics in youth work

When the first edition was published, there was very little material on ethics and values in youth work. While the literature in this field is still sparse, interest in the topic is growing and publications are beginning to emerge. In a British context, this reflects the gradual professionalisation of youth work, with qualifications for full-time youth workers now offered at degree level and a concomitant increase in youth work literature generally. It also reflects a continuing concern in all professions, and in public life, with standards of conduct and a proliferation of professional ethical codes and guidance (referred to in the first edition as the 'ethics boom'). At the time of the first edition, there was no nationally recognised code of ethics or statement of ethical principles for youth work in Britain. After consultations during 1999 to 2000 (which I coordinated), a statement was published by The National Youth Agency in 2000 covering England – which is taken into account in some of the chapters of the second edition. There have also been developments in the field of moral philosophy, with a growing literature on the ethics of character and relationship-based or 'care' ethics. These approaches to ethics are very relevant to the welfare professions, and are being increasingly developed in the literature on ethics in health and social care. While this trend was noted in the first edition, a more detailed account is offered in Chapter 1 of the new edition.

Politics in youth work

In the British political context, the period 1997 to 2010 is characterised as the 'New Labour' years – a period of Labour Party government, popularly referred to as 'New Labour' to differentiate it from the more traditional socialist orientation of the Labour Party prior to the 1990s. This government introduced a large number of very specific policies based on increasing surveillance and control over young people's lives; demands on young people to achieve qualifications and partake in training; the imposition of measurable targets for the work of professional youth work practitioners; requirements for inter-professional and inter-agency ('integrated') working; and a 'business' orientation towards public services.

While British readers (and the authors of the chapters that follow) may associate such values and policies with 'New Labour', the same broad trends have been apparent in many other Western countries (under 'neo-liberal' regimes ranging from right- to left-wing), even if the specific policies and practices may not have been quite so target-driven, measurement-oriented or marketised as in Britain. Furthermore, the ramifications of the global economic crisis that unravelled in 2008 include increasing concerns in many countries about youth unemployment and poor work opportunities, alongside policies of cutting back and restructuring welfare systems – including programmes of education, social services and leisure provision that affect young people and those who work with them.

It is hoped, therefore, that the issues discussed in this book will be of relevance to youth practitioners in a range of countries – from Iceland (where the first edition has been in use at the University of Iceland), to India (where one of the authors worked on her chapter) or the USA (where policies such as youth curfews were first developed), as well as in Britain. Despite each country having different traditions of welfare work, with different configurations and titles for the volunteers and professionally qualified practitioners who specialise in informal educational work with young people, many of the ethical dilemmas, problems and issues faced by practitioners are very similar. Examples discussed in this book include: how to challenge unjust policies and organisational norms; when to promise and when to break confidentiality; whether to exclude one young person from an activity for the benefit of others; how much weight to give to parents' and carers' views and rights when these conflict with those of a young person; when to report a young person to the police or other authorities; how much to attempt to influence young people for their own good; how much to respect young people's rights to make their own decisions and choices and to learn from their mistakes; and whether and when to intervene as an advocate on behalf of young people. These types of ethical difficulties are perennial and universal, although the ways in which they are played out, the nuances of the particular problems and dilemmas, and the language and concepts used to describe and define the issues vary between cultures and countries.

Since the chapter authors are all based in Britain (although several bring experiences from living and working in other countries), the policy and practice context in which they locate their chapters is inevitably a British one. Indeed, like all welfare practices, youth work is deeply contextualised in specific cultural, social and political settings. So to present decontextualised and abstract ethical debates about rights and responsibilities, choice and constraint, caring and controlling would distort the nature of youth work, which is about particular people living in specific places under distinctive political regimes. The aim of the book is to provide materials for ethical reflection and debate, with readers interpreting and adapting the ideas and materials to illuminate their own situations. Each chapter ends with questions for reflection in order to stimulate the thinking of individual readers and to provoke critical dialogue within groups of students and practitioners.

Content of the book

Reflecting the changes in policy and practice and developments in theory, several chapters have been completely rewritten for the second edition. These include Chapter 2, on working in welfare, which gives an overview of the British policy context (Mizen) and Chapter 6, on youth workers as moral philosophers, which develops a character-based approach to ethics (Young). Others have been substantially revised and updated, particularly Chapter 3 on ethics, collaboration and the organisational context, which now includes a new section on inter-agency working in relation to young people (McCulloch and Tett).

This edition also contains three new contributions: Chapter 5 on youth workers as professionals, covering tensions in balancing personal and professional boundaries (Sercombe); Chapter 11 on youth workers as researchers, with a particular focus on research in contexts where practitioners work (Batsleer); and Chapter 12 on young people as activists, including the issues faced by youth workers supporting young people to challenge the status quo (Wood). Readers familiar with the first edition will notice that the chapters on rights-based approaches and young people as researchers do not feature in this edition. This is not because those topics are no longer important. Rather, the theme of rights is incorporated into the new chapter (12) on young people as activists, which is based around the idea of young people as active citizens with certain rights; while the chapter on youth workers as researchers (11) includes the idea of participatory research, which involves young people as researchers.

In spite of new emphases in theory, policy and practice reflected in the chapters mentioned above, the perennial issues are solidly represented in updated chapters on the ethical issues and dilemmas associated with: resourcing youth work (Chapter 4, Jeffs and Smith); youth workers as controllers (Chapter 7, Jeffs and Banks); youth workers as converters in faith-based settings (Chapter 8, Green); youth workers as mediators in work with black young people (Chapter 9, Imam and Bowler); and youth workers as confidants in contexts where the welfare and safety of young people or others may compromise confidentiality or where inter-agency working challenges the youth work relationship (Chapter 10, Morgan and Banks). Chapter 1 offers a short introduction to the topic of ethics and youth work, discussing the contested nature of youth work and a range of theoretical approaches to ethics.

Part 1
The ethical context of youth work

<table>
<tr><td>1</td></tr>
</table>

Ethics and the youth worker

Sarah Banks

Introduction

Case study 1.1

While out on a trip with a group of young people, I [a female youth worker] saw one of the participants, a young woman, stealing sweets from a shop. Nobody else seemed to have noticed. The young woman had recently returned to the youth club following a long absence and her behaviour was often challenging. I felt I was just beginning to develop a relationship of trust with her, and therefore decided not to mention the theft. Afterwards I wondered if I had done the right thing: by not mentioning the incident, I was condoning the theft and passing on the value that it was acceptable.

This case was given as an example of an ethical dilemma by a female student studying youth and community work in Britain. It is an account of an everyday incident, probably remembered because the youth worker at the time was relatively inexperienced and questioned whether her response was the right one. All youth workers can give examples of similar incidents and dilemmas – of cases where they have had to make a difficult choice about what to do, and wondered afterwards if what they did was right.

Ethical issues are endemic in youth work. As an activity or practice, youth work involves working with participants who have fewer rights than adults, are often vulnerable, lack power and may be suggestible – hence giving scope for their exploitation, harm or manipulation. As an occupation working within the welfare system, youth work shares with social work, nursing and medicine the classic tensions between respecting individual choice and promoting the public good; and between empowering and controlling its service users. Like social work, it has to work within societal ambivalence towards its service users (young people are often regarded as threatening or undeserving) – balancing the roles of carer, protector, advocate and liberator. Insofar as it is an occupation concerned with providing a service, youth work shares with a broad group of occupations, commonly classed as professions, concerns about the professional integrity, trustworthiness and honesty of its practitioners.

These features of youth work suggest that there is plenty of scope for examining and debating the ethical issues, problems and dilemmas that arise in practice. In setting the scene for the rest of the book, this chapter will examine the nature of youth work and consider debates about the boundaries of the work and its status as a 'profession'. It will then consider what we mean by 'ethics', briefly distinguishing two broad theoretical approaches to ethics and their implications for professional ethics in a youth work context.

The nature of youth work

'What is youth work?' is a perennial question debated among practitioners and in the literature. To answer the question I will first examine different uses of the term 'youth work' before discussing its substantive nature (purpose, values and activities).

The concept of 'youth work'

'Youth work' is used in several different ways. It may describe: (1) an activity or practice (what people do); (2) an occupation (a practice undertaken by qualified or recognised workers within a culture of norms); and (3) a discipline (an identifiable area of study and practice) – as summarised in List 1.1.

List 1.1: Three senses of 'youth work'

1 **Youth work as an activity (work with young people).** 'Youth work' in this broad sense describes a range of different types of work with young people undertaken by volunteers and people professionally qualified in a variety of professions or disciplines, including:

   a) *Generic work with young people using a range of approaches and purposes.* This is a wide category covering the practices of school teaching, police work with young people, social work with young people and sports coaching, for example, as well as specialist youth work undertaken by youth workers.

b) *Work with young people with an informal educational and/or developmental focus.* This is a slightly more specialist category of work that takes into account the approach to the work and its purpose (informal education and/or personal and social development). The work may be undertaken by paid workers (sometimes professionally qualified) or volunteers. 'Informal education' entails young people learning through participation in activities; 'personal and social development' has a more specific focus on young people maturing and taking roles as responsible citizens. This category may include the work of teachers when taking young people on a sporting trip or police officers when working with a group of young people on the theme of knife crime, as well as the work of specialist youth workers in a youth project or club.

2   **Youth work as a specialist occupation.** This describes work with young people with an informal educational and/or developmental approach and purpose that is carried out by people who are qualified as youth workers, or who consciously adopt the identity of 'youth worker' within an organisational setting (this includes volunteers and part-time workers).

3   **Youth work as a discipline.** This refers to a body of theory and practice that can be taught, learnt and studied (e.g. mathematics or geography), as well as practised. Youth work as a discipline develops from and influences the activities and practices of youth work as an occupation. If students say they are studying 'youth work' at university, this is what they mean.

It could be argued that the first category (youth work as an activity) should not be called 'youth work' at all. Rather it should be referred to as 'work with young people' to avoid confusion with youth work as a specialist occupation and youth work as a discipline. I have included this meaning of 'youth work' since the term is sometimes used in this broad way – especially in international contexts. Nevertheless, the concern in this book is largely with the activities and practices undertaken within *youth work as a specialist occupation*. Although many of the ethical issues and dilemmas are relevant to all those who work with young people and will be of interest to practitioners in a range of fields, the examples given and contexts described focus largely on the work of specialist youth workers. However, lines are difficult to draw. Problems of identity and definition are compounded by the fact that 'youth work' is not internationally recognised as a specialist occupation (and certainly not as a profession) in the way that medicine, law, architecture, nursing or social work tend to be, with international professional associations and codes of ethics.

Varieties of youth work

In most countries youth work includes the work of volunteers in independent (that is, not state-run) youth organisations (such as the scouts and guides, boys' brigades, girls' clubs and religious youth movements) as well as the work of volunteers and paid workers in more professionalised statutory or not-for-profit youth services and programmes (such as local authority children's and young people's services; youth projects run by Save the Children or the St Vincent de Paul Society). However, the ways in which the more professionalised services are organised and the nature of the professional identities and education of the people who staff these services are very varied. In some countries paid work with young people with an informal educational focus is undertaken within an occupational group known as 'youth work' with specialist education and training – for example, Britain and Australia. Elsewhere the paid work is done by pedagogues (for example, Belgium, Denmark or Germany), specialised educators (such as in France), youth development workers (USA) or distributed among social workers, community workers or leisure workers.

The way in which job titles and organisational configurations vary between different countries and even within countries (linked to continually developing social policies and welfare systems) has led some commentators to speak of the 'identity crisis' of youth work. Verschelden *et al.* (2009: 4) nevertheless note that among contributors at a European seminar on the history of youth work in 2008, it was possible to identify some key characteristics of youth work across countries and over time as follows:

- being young together;
- often, but not always, with a shared ideology or project;
- nurturing associational life;
- providing opportunities for social contact, recreation and education.

However, this is a very generic set of characteristics, which captures the second part (b) of the first category of youth work as an activity, but is not specific enough to be a set of defining features of youth work as an occupation or discipline. It could apply, for example, to the work of a schoolteacher on a school trip or a police officer running a youth football team.

Baizerman (1996, quoted in Coussée 2008: 6) urges against seeking a single model of youth work that might be valid worldwide, instead referring to youth work as a 'family of practices'. If we develop this idea in accordance with the philosopher Wittgenstein's (1972: par. 67) account of 'family resemblances', this implies that there is no single feature or set of features that may be regarded as essentially defining 'youth work'. Rather there may be family resemblances and overlapping characteristics between different activities and practices we call 'youth work'. For example, while the majority of youth work activities and projects have

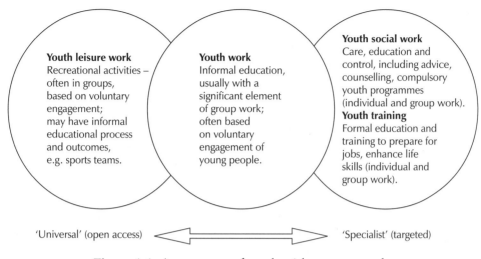

Youth leisure work
Recreational activities –
often in groups,
based on voluntary
engagement;
may have informal
educational process
and outcomes,
e.g. sports teams.

Youth work
Informal education,
usually with a
significant element
of group work;
often based
on voluntary
engagement of
young people.

Youth social work
Care, education and
control, including advice,
counselling, compulsory
youth programmes
(individual and group work).
Youth training
Formal education and
training to prepare for
jobs, enhance life
skills (individual and
group work).

'Universal' (open access) ⟵⟶ 'Specialist' (targeted)

Figure 1.1 A spectrum of work with young people

an informal educational focus at their core, some may have as a primary purpose the control of young people, formal training or the provision of leisure activities. Much youth work is centred around work with groups of young people, but there are some youth work projects that are solely casework or individual focused. Many activities classed as 'youth work' are based on the voluntary engagement of young people, but some rely on compulsory referrals from courts or social services. Figure 1.1 is an attempt to show in a schematic way a continuum of work with young people, illustrating how what is called 'youth work' as an occupation overlaps with a range of leisure, formal education and control activities and practices.

However, there are some youth work theorists and practitioners who would argue that there *are* defining features of youth work and if an activity or practice does not have certain features (such as an educational purpose, group work and voluntary engagement), then it is not youth work (Davies 2005; Jeffs and Smith 2008). This could be termed an essentialist view, which, if taken literally, results in a very narrow definition of youth work (Payne 2009). Such a definition either excludes much of what is currently labelled as 'youth work' from being regarded as 'true youth work' (ignoring the overlaps in the concentric circles in Figure 1.1) or magnifies the disjunction between 'ideal youth work' and 'youth work in reality'. This gap between ideal and reality may be viewed as indicative of youth work's immaturity and inconsistency, and as providing evidence of an identity crisis. However, it might be more useful to view the essentialist account of youth work not in terms of an immutable set of (unrealistic) defining characteristics, but rather as what Weber (1978) calls an 'ideal type'. Freidson (2001) uses this concept in his study of professions in general. In the context of youth work, this would entail producing a list of characteristics of 'ideal-typical' youth work in order to provide a standard against which to evaluate historical and current activities and occupations whose characteristics vary according to time and place. It enables us to judge activities and occupations against the ideal-type, without claiming that the ideal-type describes any real occupation or set of activities.

Fixing youth work: the British example

As some of the activities and practices associated with youth work have become recognised as forming an occupation and as providing the subject matter for an applied academic discipline, sets of standards and benchmarks have been developed that begin to 'fix' its characteristics. Taking Britain as an example, as part of a broader project to standardise qualifications across the whole 'vocational' workforce, which started with national vocational qualifications in the 1990s (Banks 1996), there are now national occupational standards for youth work (Lifelong Learning UK 2008). These lay out the purpose and values of youth work and the abilities required by qualified youth workers to undertake a range of defined functional activities. They are used as a framework for professional qualifying education and training and as a guide for employers in drawing up job descriptions and staff development programmes. In 2000 a statement on *Ethical Conduct in Youth Work* was published by The National Youth Agency, which covers England. Although The National Youth Agency has no powers to enforce the principles outlined in the statement, and there is no professional association or professional registration council for all qualified youth workers, this statement nevertheless partly fulfils the role of a code of professional ethics in guiding and educating practitioners and employers (Banks 2003a). In relation to youth work as discipline, higher education subject benchmarks have been produced covering 'youth and community work' (Quality Assurance Agency 2009) for which the professional qualification level will be at Bachelor's degree level from 2010. This benchmark statement reflects youth work's historic association with community work, which is still maintained in the content of professional education programmes.

The creation of standards, principles and benchmarks exemplifies a slow move towards the definition and recognition of youth work as a distinctive occupation and an academic discipline in Britain, and may be used in the creation of an ideal-type for youth work. To some extent these trends are moves towards 'professionalisation', insofar as this entails the development of a distinct occupational identity, a set of values and increased levels of education and qualification. Yet they do not necessarily entail other features commonly associated with professionalisation, such as: a high degree of autonomy by practitioners over how they do their work; a strong community of practitioners belonging to professional associations with power and influence over entry to the occupation; or nationally recognised systems for the registration (licensing) and deregistration of practitioners (Koehn 1994). However, rather than focusing on key traits of professions or the power of professional elites, it may be more helpful to adopt a historical/developmental approach to the study of professions (Siegrist 1994). This entails looking at the changing patterns of occupational groups over time, between locations and in relation to political and policy contexts (Banks 2004; Freidson 2001). The story of the development of youth work must be located in the context of various moral panics about young people, and the social policies and political configurations of particular times and places, as some of the historical accounts of youth work written to date clearly exemplify (Coussée 2008; Davies 1999a, 1999b, 2008; Jeffs 1979).

Although definitive statements about the purpose, nature and values of youth work have been produced in various manifestos, policy documents, academic books and articles, youth workers on the ground continue to experience and voice uncertainty about identities, roles and values (Spence *et al.* 2007; Tucker 2004). This can be explained by the natural gap between ideal-type and reality that is felt by all professions. Furthermore, the gap may be wider than in many other occupations, as youth work is a small grouping without strong professional bodies to promote and defend it. Youth workers can easily be diverted or co-opted to tackling the latest moral panic or centrally defined targets for crime reduction or teenage pregnancy (see Chapter 7, this volume). In such cases, relationships with young people may be a means to the end of changing behaviour or contributing to the achievement of a government target rather than a good in itself or a good for the young people concerned. Increasing requirements for multi- and inter-professional working in integrated services generate fears that the distinctive youth work identity, role and values may be lost. The demands outlined in recent English policy (see Mizen, Chapter 2, this volume) are for a flexible, joined-up and interchangeable children's and youth workforce, members of which can join hands to surround, support, control and contain young people individually and in groups. Although it may be argued that the youth work role and youth workers' identities can and should be strengthened in such contexts (Banks 2004: 125–148, 2009), this requires a level of clarity and confidence on the part of youth workers and their managers that does not always materialise.

While the written statements of purpose and values in themselves cannot defend youth workers from being co-opted to controlling or casework roles, they do provide invaluable 'lighthouses' (Clark 1999) or 'beacons' that may be used as reference points in times of darkness or when there is a feeling that the occupation is losing its way. If we examine the many recent British and English statements outlining the core purpose of youth work, the values upon which it is based and the commitments required of youth workers, despite some differences in wording and emphasis, there is remarkable consensus. List 1.2 offers a summary, drawing upon a range of sources. The key purpose is taken verbatim from the national occupational standards for youth work (LLUK 2008). The values draw upon Davies (2005), DfES (2002), LLUK (2008) and Taylor (2009). The youth workers' commitments are modified from *Ethical Conduct in Youth Work* (NYA 2000). The first four commitments comprise the ethical principles, with the fifth commitment consolidating the four professional principles listed in the NYA statement, following Banks (2009).

List 1.2: The purpose, values and ethical principles of youth work – an ideal-type

The key purpose of youth work is to:

Enable young people to develop holistically, working with them to facilitate their personal, social and educational development, to enable them to develop their voice, influence and place in society and to reach their full potential.

Youth work has the following characteristics and values:

- A *voluntary relationship* with young people, who are free to choose whether or not to be involved.
- An *informal educational process* that starts where young people are starting, and seeks to go beyond where young people start by encouraging them to be outward-looking, critical and creative in their responses to their experiences and the world around them.
- *The value of association*, which involves young people working together in groups, fostering supportive relationships and sharing a common life.
- *The value of young people participating democratically* and as fully as possible in making decisions about issues that affect them in youth work contexts and in life generally.

Youth workers have a commitment to the following ethical principles:

1. *Respect young people*, recognising and valuing each young person's identity, emotions and capabilities and avoiding adult-imposed labels and negative discrimination.
2. *Respect and promote young people's rights to make their own decisions and choices*, unless the welfare or legitimate interests of themselves or others are seriously threatened. This includes working towards the empowerment of young people to have a voice and to influence the environment in which they live.
3. *Promote and ensure the welfare and safety of young people*, while permitting them to learn through undertaking challenging educational activities.
4. *Contribute towards the promotion of social justice for young people and in society generally*, through encouraging respect for difference and diversity, recognising the influences of class, gender, ethnicity, sexuality and ability and challenging discrimination.

5   *Practise with integrity, compassion, courage and competence*, which includes: being honest and open in dealings with young people; not exploiting relationships; recognising boundaries between personal and professional life; managing multiple professional accountabilities; maintaining competence required for the job; fostering ethical debate; working for conditions in employing agencies so that the values of youth work are upheld; and being prepared to challenge colleagues and employers in breach of these values.

Such statements of purpose and values remain contestable and open to change. Some practitioners and academics may disagree with some parts of them. However, in times of challenge and change, it is important that youth workers are familiar with these statements and are prepared to use them when employers, colleagues, other professionals, agencies or members of the public make inappropriate or even unethical demands. The account given in Chapter 10 (Case study 10.4) about police officers asking youth workers for details of young people filmed by security cameras is just such an example. While lists of values and ethical principles do not provide direct guidance to workers about how to act in particular cases, they do serve as a reminder of the kinds of values and principles upon which youth work is based and serve to encourage youth workers to think through, discuss and reflect on the implications of their decisions and actions.

The nature of ethics

Having considered the nature of youth work, we will now explore what is meant by 'ethics'. In English the term has a plural and a singular meaning. I will use the term 'ethics' (plural) to refer to principles and norms of behaviour people espouse and follow in relation to right and wrong action and the good and bad qualities of character and relationships people develop that are relevant to the flourishing of human beings, animals and the planet.[1] 'Ethics' (singular) is the *study* of these principles, norms, qualities and relationships (in this sense 'ethics' is sometimes used synonymously with 'moral philosophy'). In ordinary English usage, the term 'ethics' (plural) is often used interchangeably with 'morals'. They are two words with different origins (Greek and Latin) with very similar original meanings (habits or customs). Although some theorists (especially in the continental European literature) do distinguish between ethics as internally generated norms and morals as externally generated prevailing societal norms (Bouquet 1999; Osborne 1998), in this book the terms 'ethics' and 'ethical' are used interchangeably with 'morals' and 'moral'.

Ethics in youth work

In order to explore ethics in youth work, I will return to the Case study (1.1) presented at the start of the chapter (about the youth worker who witnessed a theft by a young person). I will identify some of the features that make it an 'ethics case', as illustrated in the following analysis.

- *Ethical issues relating human welfare and flourishing are embodied in the case.* 'Ethical issues' encompass matters of rights, duties, needs, interests, relationships, motives and the maintenance or transgression of prevailing norms. In this case, the ethical issues include the interests and needs of the young woman, who has been experiencing difficulties with her life; the interests and rights of the shopkeeper, whose goods have been stolen; the public good, which is about maintaining honesty as a prevailing norm; and the quality of the trusting relationship between the young person and the youth worker.
- A *difficult ethical decision is at stake.* By 'difficult ethical decision' is meant a problem or dilemma relating to human or animal welfare or planetary flourishing involving a choice about courses of action. Ethical problems and dilemmas may be distinguished as follows (Banks 2003b: 13–14, 2006: 103–104):
  - *an ethical problem* occurs when a difficult decision has to be made, but the person making the decision is clear about what course of action should be taken;
  - *an ethical dilemma* occurs when a person is confronted with a choice between two (or several) alternative courses of action, all of which may entail breaching some ethical principle or causing some potential harm.

  In this case, the youth worker experienced her choice as a dilemma between preserving a relationship and rectifying a theft. Although she chose the former as her preferred course of action for the reasons she outlines, this leaves her with the responsibility for not having dealt with the theft.

- A *process of ethical reflection has occurred.* Ethical reflection is a process of mulling over, questioning and appraising a matter relating to human, animal or planetary flourishing. This process may occur during an incident or activity ('reflection in action', which may be tacit or intuitive) or afterwards ('reflection on action') – to use a distinction made by Schön (1991) in his work on the reflective practitioner. In her account of the incident, the youth worker included her reflections afterwards about whether she had 'done the right thing'. Often, if the decision has involved a dilemma, there may be an element of regret or remorse – the 'moral remainder' left over when a difficult choice has been made for which there was no easy right answer (Banks and Williams 2005; Foot 2002: 175–188). The youth worker's reflections on the implications of her actions in this case exemplify this feature of ethical dilemmas.

- *Professional responsibilities are involved.* Responsibilities attach to the professional role over and above the responsibilities we might expect in everyday life (see Koehn 1994; also Sercombe, Chapter 5, this volume). In this case, the youth worker is responsible for the good behaviour of the young people in her care; for their moral education and for modelling good practice. This case is not just about ethics, but about *professional* ethics – that is, the special obligations taken on, relationships developed and qualities required by a person in a work role.

Theoretical approaches to ethics

We will now consider what theoretical resources might be available to help youth workers recognise, understand, act on and engage in dialogue about ethical issues. The literature in moral philosophy and the specialist area of professional ethics is extensive, so this brief overview is necessarily selective and simplified. I will briefly outline two types of theoretical approach to ethics and their implications for professional ethics in youth work: principle-based approaches, and character- and relationship-based approaches, relating them to Case study 1.1 and to the list of features of ideal-typical youth work (List 1.2).

Principle-based approaches to ethics

Until recently, much of the Anglo-American literature on ethics in the welfare and caring field has tended to focus on the identification, interpretation and implementation of the core ethical principles of particular professions. The principles are often discussed in the context of two different ethical traditions – Kantianism and utilitarianism – both of which have at their heart the notion of the individual moral agent as a rational decision-maker (for a more detailed discussion see Banks 2006: 27–53).

Immanual Kant, an eighteenth-century German philosopher (1724–1804), developed a theory of ethics based on the ultimate principle of respect for the individual person (Kant 1785/1964). This approach to ethics, often termed 'deontological' or duty-based, has been very influential in moral philosophy and also in professional ethics. 'Persons' are regarded as rational and self-determining – that is, capable of making choices and acting upon them. Kantian ethics in a professional context tends to focus on respect for and promotion of the autonomy of the service user and would stress principles such as maintaining confidentiality, obtaining informed consent, not acting in a stigmatising or discriminatory manner or offering misleading or untruthful information. For Kant, any action that violated the principle of respect for persons would be morally wrong – regardless of whether it resulted in an outcome viewed as beneficial. For example, if a youth worker lied to a threatening father about the whereabouts of his son, this would be wrong, regardless of the fact that the lie was told to protect the young man from being beaten up. The youth worker in Case study 1.1, by remaining silent, was failing to treat the young woman with respect, as a free, rational and responsible agent, able to take responsibility for her actions. Although the youth worker did not lie to the young women, it could be argued she was being dishonest in not communicating her disapproval about the theft. The ethical principles in List 1.2 relating to respecting young people (1) and respecting their choices (2) could be described as 'Kantian' principles.

Utilitarianism, on the other hand, is a teleological or consequentialist theory of ethics, particularly associated with two British philosophers, Jeremy Bentham (1748–1832) and John Stuart Mill (1806–1873) (Mill 1863/1972). In contrast to Kantian ethics, the moral worth (rightness or wrongness) of an action is said to lie in its consequences; hence deciding what is right involves anticipating, weighing up and balancing the consequences. Many versions of utilitarianism have been developed, but the basic idea is very simple: that the right action is that which produces the greatest balance of good over evil (the principle of utility). Thus, for example, if lying would produce good consequences overall, then lying would be right. In the case of the youth worker asked by a threatening father to reveal where his son is, telling a lie might be regarded as morally right if, in weighing up the consequences of telling the truth or lying, the youth worker decided that more harm would be done if the truth were told. Core principles for professional workers relate to the promotion of the welfare of service users, the promotion of the greater good in society and the distribution of goods in a fair and just manner. It is recognised that the question of 'whose good?' is an important one, which is where the principle of justice comes in, that the good should be as widely distributed as possible; that is, the right action is that which produces the greatest good for the greatest number of people. Philosophers have disagreed over what counts as good: whether it is just pleasure or happiness, or it includes virtue, knowledge and truth. The ethical principles in List 1.2 about promoting welfare (3) and contributing to social justice (4) could be regarded as utilitarian principles.

Criticisms may be levelled at both Kantian and utilitarian systems of ethical thinking, especially if they are regarded as mutually exclusive ethical theories designed to capture the whole of moral life. For the purposes of this discussion it is sufficient to note that people do seem to take account of both types of ethical principles in making decisions. Some of the most difficult choices and dilemmas relate to tensions between respecting individual freedom and rights, and promoting the welfare of an individual or a larger group of people in society. Even the relatively minor dilemma in Case study 1.1 about whether to tackle the young woman about the theft of the sweets could be interpreted as exemplifying the tensions between the youth worker treating the young woman honestly (a Kantian principle) by confronting her openly about what she had done; and protecting or promoting her welfare (a utilitarian principle) by not disturbing the relationship.

Character- and relationship-based ethics

Principle-based ethical theories such as Kantianism and utilitarianism have been subject to a range of critiques in recent years. They present the core ethical principles as universal, applying to all people at all times and in all places, assuming ethics as being about rational and impartial decision-making in weighing up which principles to prioritise and deriving more specific rules or ethical standards from the general principles. They ignore important features of moral life and moral judgements, including the character, motives and emotions of the people making the decisions and taking action, the particular contexts in which judgements are made and the specific commitments and relationships people have with each other. Principle-based ethics is often described as very Western in outlook, valuing individual choice and freedom, and downplaying the importance of communal commitments and relationships that might be predominant in non-Western societies, cultures and religions (see Imam and Bowler, Chapter 9, this volume). I will now briefly outline two approaches to ethics that are more situated and contextual: virtue ethics (which focuses on the character of the moral agent) and the ethics of care (which focuses on relationships).

Virtue ethics is associated with the ancient Greek philosopher, Aristotle (384–322 BC), although there are many other versions, including a recent revival of interest in virtue ethics (Aristotle 1954 edition; Hursthouse 1999; MacIntyre 1985; Swanton 2003; Van Hooft 2006). What they have in common is a focus on people's character or dispositions as opposed to abstract obligations, duties or principles for action. One of the reasons suggested for the growing popularity of virtue ethics is that principles are too abstract to provide helpful guidance in the complicated situations met in everyday life. Virtues also seem to provide a more commonly accepted currency for talking about ethics across cultures and religions. Virtue ethics is an approach 'according to which the basic judgements in ethics are judgements about character' (Statman 1997: 7). In Hursthouse's version of virtue ethics, an action is right if it is what a virtuous agent would do in the circumstances; a virtue is 'a character trait a human being needs to flourish or live well' (Hursthouse 1997: 229). What counts as 'living well' or 'flourishing' then becomes an important question in deciding what characteristics count as virtues. Some virtue theorists argue that these vary according to different time periods and cultures (for example, the kinds of characteristics cultivated as virtues in ancient Greece may not all be applicable in twenty-first-century Europe, Africa or Asia); others claim that there are universal virtues. Nevertheless, the kinds of dispositions usually regarded as virtues include courage, integrity, honesty, truthfulness, loyalty, wisdom and kindness, for example. A virtuous person will give an honest response to a question, it would be argued, not because of some abstract principle stating 'you shall not lie', or because on this occasion telling the truth will produce a good result, but because that person does not want to be the sort of person who tells lies. In the case of the threatening father asking the youth worker to reveal the whereabouts of his son, the youth worker with a disposition towards honesty might engage in a conversation with the father to explain his professional role in relation to protecting the young man and why he is not able to reveal his whereabouts.

Young (Chapter 6, this volume) offers a virtue-based approach to ethics in youth work, reflecting a growing interest in virtues in the field of professional ethics (Banks and Gallagher 2008; Oakley and Cocking 2001). The fifth commitment in List 1.2 is, in effect, a list of virtues, outlining the kind of person a good youth worker should be (for example, honest and courageous). The youth worker in Case study 1.1 would probably develop these qualities over time and with experience, so that in similar situations in the future she might engage in constructive conversations with young people who steal or commit other misdemeanours.

There are a number of critiques of virtue ethics, including the argument that lists of virtues are just as abstract and unhelpful in making everyday ethical decisions as are lists of values or ethical principles. Some philosophers have actually argued that virtue ethics can be subsumed within principle-based ethics – for example, that being a fair person simply consists in a disposition to act fairly – and therefore our moral judgements must be grounded in judgements about people's actions rather than their characters.

Virtue ethics has also been criticised for focusing particularly on 'male' virtues (such as courage) while ignoring those that are needed to help others (such as care or compassion). This critique is countered by ethical theories that focus on care as the core of ethics. This type of approach to ethics has been associated particularly, although not exclusively, with modern feminist philosophers. Some philosophers have developed an ethics of care as a form of virtue ethics, seeing care as a core virtue (Slote 2007; Van Hooft 2006), while others have developed an approach to ethics that sees care as a relation, rather than a virtue (Held 2006; Noddings 1984, 2002). Recent developments of a relational ethics of care owe much to the empirical work of psychologist Carol Gilligan (1982) who identified two 'moral voices' in her interviews with people about how they conceptualised and spoke about moral dilemmas. She contrasts the 'ethic of care' with what she calls the 'ethic of justice'. The ethic of justice refers to principle-based approaches to ethics, based on a system of individualised rights and duties, emphasising abstract moral principles, impartiality and rationality. Gilligan argues that this fails to take account of approaches to ethics that tend to be adopted by women, which would emphasise responsibility rather than duty and relationships rather than principles. Furthermore, as Tronto (1993) argues, the ethics of care, with its stress on relationship and responsibility, fits better with the cultural and religious norms of many societies in the global South. Gilligan herself is equivocal about the extent to which an ethic of care should be regarded as a 'female' or 'feminine' ethics, although some care ethicists do explicitly adopt this point of view.

Case study 1.1 is a good example of a youth worker regarding a relationship with a particular young person as a key element in her ethical decision-making and actions. However, while prioritising a relationship with a known young woman over justice for an unknown shopkeeper might seem on the face of it to be a response consistent with the ethics of care, arguably a more genuine relationship of care might have been maintained and developed through engaging in a dialogue with the young woman about her behaviour in the shop. Tronto (1993: 127–136) develops an account of the elements of care, which comprise not only caring about the other person (awareness of the other and her needs), but taking care of the other person (assuming responsibility for care) and care-giving (the ability to do something about the other's needs). A caring relationship between a youth worker and a young person entails more than the youth worker simply caring about the young person; it entails caring for the young person responsibly. Nevertheless, an ethic of care seems inadequate on its own as an account of professional ethics (Banks 2004: 70–105; Kuhse 1997). The emphasis on the unique caring relationship and responsibility of the care-giver can be dangerous in professional life, where impartiality is important and there is a danger in taking too much responsibility for the well-being of others. Caring relationships can be suffocating and controlling as well as enriching and empowering.

The importance of principles, character and relationships

This account of a variety of theoretical approaches suggests that no single ethical theory adequately encompasses all features of what we want to include as the subject matter of ethics. Arguably an ethics of character and relationships that takes into account people's motives and moral qualities, the particularity of each situation, people's relationships with each other, cooperation, communication and caring is important and complementary to an ethics of principle that stresses universal principles of individual freedom, justice, social contracts and duty. An excessive emphasis in professional ethics on the latter may result in over-regulation, a damaging impartiality and neutrality, and a mindless following of rules for their own sake. As Baier (1995: 48) comments, justice is found to be too 'cold' and 'it is "warmer" more communitarian virtues and social ideals that are being called in to supplement it'. Yet, at the same time, in the delivery of publicly funded and organised services, universally applicable rules are an important part of what defines the work of the professionals delivering these services. Professional workers are not expected to give preferential treatment to their neighbour's daughter over and above a stranger, for example, although they may do so in everyday life. Approaches to ethics based on character and relationships and approaches based on principles are not mutually exclusive; they are, as Mendus

(1993: 18) argues, 'complementary facets of any realistic account of morality'. List 1.3 summarises key features of these theoretical approaches, all of which need to form the basis of a comprehensive framework for understanding professional ethics (see also Banks and Imam 2000)

List 1.3: Approaches to professional ethics[2]

1   Principle-based ethics

  a) 'Kantian' principles, for example:

  - respect for persons;
  - self-determination of service users;
  - respect for confidentiality.

  b) Utilitarian principles, for example:

  - promotion of welfare/goods;
  - just distribution of welfare/goods.

2   Character- and relationship-based ethics

  a) Virtue ethics – development of character/virtues/excellences, such as:

  - honesty;
  - compassion;
  - professional integrity.

  b) Ethics of care – importance of particular relationships, involving:

  - care;
  - attentiveness;
  - responsibility.

Elements of ethics in professional life

I will now return again to Case study 1.1 to elucidate these points further. By reflecting on this relatively commonplace and apparently simple example, the complexities of ethical and practical understandings, attitudes, decision-making and actions become apparent. Ethics is often presented as being about making difficult choices in situations where several (apparently universal) ethical principles are in conflict – in this case, promoting honesty versus promoting an individual's welfare. However, there are other important ingredients in a case such as this, of which I will highlight three, that link to virtues and caring relationships as well as to principles and reasoning.

1 *Ethical sensitivity.* First, a situation or occurrence has to be perceived as one where ethical issues are at stake – for example, where there is an infringement of rights, a case of potential harm or a call for a response. This requires not only knowledge of abstract principles, but sensitivity to the nuances of situations and a relational capacity for empathy and moral imagination (linked to an ethics of care). In Case study 1.1 the worker was clearly sensitive to the psychological state of the young woman, as well as recognising that the young woman had acted wrongly.

2 *Ethical reasoning.* A process of ethical reasoning may take place, although this may be imperfect and constrained by time in the immediacy of a particular event. This involves assessing the nature of the situation and the duties involved; weighing up different principles and courses of action; calculating harms and benefits; and deciding what is the right course of action (linked to principle-based ethics). In Case study 1.1 the worker had already made a decision about what to do and gave her reason (that the relationship of trust with the young woman was vulnerable). Her account of herself wondering afterwards if what she did was right was a further continuation of a process of reasoning that was probably incomplete and unclear at the time of the incident.

3 *Qualities of character and competence.* Even if a clear ethical evaluation has been made about what is the right course of action, whether and how this is implemented will be influenced by the moral and practical qualities of the person concerned. The person may lack the courage or commitment to do what they know is right (linked to virtue ethics); or they may feel that they do not have the skills or knowledge. In Case study 1.1 we might surmise that perhaps the worker was not experienced, skilled or courageous enough to engage honestly with the young woman. As part of the process of talking through her example, and undertaking professional education, she might develop her competence, confidence and courage.

Conclusion

In this chapter I have used one example of a relatively simple, everyday ethical dilemma to elucidate the nature of ethics and offer an account of various components of ethical seeing, being and doing in a youth work context. Other chapters in this volume address more complex ethical difficulties, involving, for example, risks of serious harm, racism and inter-cultural, inter-agency and inter-professional conflicts where youth workers' clarity of moral purpose, qualities of character and commitments to the core ethical principles of youth work are vital. Hopefully the ethical framework offered here will be equally useful in a range of contexts to facilitate critical ethical reflection, analysis and dialogue.

Questions for reflection and discussion

1 Think of an ethical problem or dilemma you have experienced in your personal or professional life. What ethical principles were at stake? What responsibilities and relationships did you and the other participants have? What qualities of character did you and other participants exhibit or lack? What did you do and how would you justify your course of action ethically?

2 Study the values and ethical principles given in List 1.1. Do you agree with them? Would you modify the list?

3 What do you think are the most important moral qualities of character for youth workers and why?

Recommended reading

Banks, S. (2009) 'Values and ethics in work with young people', in J. Hine and J. Wood (eds) *Work with Young People: Developments in Theory, Policy and Practice*, London: Sage. This chapter introduces the concept of values in youth work and explores in detail a particular example of an ethically challenging situation experienced by a youth worker in a youth offending team.

Banks, S. and Gallagher, A. (2008) *Ethics in Professional Life: Virtues for Health and Social Care*, Basingstoke: Palgrave Macmillan. This book develops a virtue-based approach to professional ethics with a particular focus on health and social care. It has chapters on key virtues such as courage, justice, care, integrity and trustworthiness, which are also relevant to youth work.

Boss, J. (2007) *Ethics for Life: A Text with Readings*, 3rd edition, New York, McGraw-Hill. This book gives useful background information on various ethical theories and is written in a clear, practical style. It includes photographs/drawings of key thinkers and their biographical details, and includes discussion of religion and cultural relativism.

Acknowledgements

I am very grateful to a youth worker for allowing me to use material relating to an ethical dilemma in her practice.

Notes

1 I have used the term 'flourishing' instead of 'well-being' or 'welfare' in order to encompass environmental sustainability within the subject matter of ethics. 'Flourishing' is a contested concept, normally associated with virtue ethics, with connotations of wholeness, living well and fulfilling a purpose.
2 This list is a modified version taken from Banks (2001: 4).

References

Aristotle (1954 edition) *The Nichomachean Ethics of Aristotle, Translated by Sir David Ross*, London: Oxford University Press.

Baier, A. (1995) 'The need for more than justice', in V. Held (ed.) *Justice and Care: Essential Readings in Feminist Ethics*, Boulder, CO: Westview Press.

Baizerman, M. (1996) 'Youth work on the street. Community's moral compact with its young people', *Childhood*, 3: 157–165.

Banks, S. (1996) 'Youth work, informal education and professionalisation: the issues in the 1990s', *Youth and Policy*, 54: 13–25.

Banks, S. (2001) 'Ethical dilemmas for the social professions: work in progress with social education students in Europe', *European Journal of Social Education*, 1: 1–16.

Banks, S. (2003a) 'From oaths to rulebooks: a critical examination of codes of ethics for the social professions', *European Journal of Social Work*, 6: 133–144.

Banks, S. (2003b) 'Conflicts of culture and accountability: managing ethical dilemmas and problems in community practice', in S. Banks, H. Butcher, P. Henderson and J. Robertson (eds) *Managing Community Practice: Principles, Policies and Programmes*, Bristol: Policy Press.

Banks, S. (2004) *Ethics, Accountability and the Social Professions*, Basingstoke: Palgrave Macmillan.

Banks, S. (2006) *Ethics and Values in Social Work*, 3rd edn, Basingstoke: Palgrave Macmillan.

Banks, S. (2009) 'Values and ethics in work with young people', in J. Hine and J. Wood (eds) *Work with Young People: Developments in Theory, Policy and Practice*, London: Sage.

Banks, S. and Gallagher, A. (2008) *Ethics in Professional Life: Virtues for Health and Social Care*, Basingstoke: Palgrave Macmillan.

Banks, S. and Imam, U. (2000) 'Principles, rules and qualities: an ethical framework for youth work', *International Journal of Adolescence and Youth*, 9: 61–78.

Banks, S. and Williams, R. (2005) 'Accounting for ethical difficulties in social welfare work: issues, problems and dilemmas', *British Journal of Social Work*, 35: 1005–1022.

Bouquet, B. (1999) 'De l'éthique personelle à une éthique professionelle', *EMPAN*, 36: 27–33.

Clark, C. (1999) 'Observing the lighthouse: from theory to institutions in social work ethics', *European Journal of Social Work*, 2: 259–270.

Coussée, F. (2008) *A Century of Youth Work Policy*, Gent: Academia Press.

Davies, B. (1999a) *From Voluntaryism to Welfare State: A History of the Youth Service in England, Volume 1, 1939–1979*, Leicester: Youth Work Press.

Davies, B. (1999b) *From Thatcherism to New Labour: A History of the Youth Service in England, Volume 2, 1979–1999*, Leicester: Youth Work Press.

Davies, B. (2005) 'Youth work: a manifesto for our times', *Youth and Policy*, 88: 5–27.

Davies, B. (2008) *The New Labour Years: A History of the Youth Service in England, Volume 3, 199[7]–2007*, Leicester: The National Youth Agency.

Department for Education and Skills (DfES) (2002) *Transforming Youth Work: Resourcing Excellent Youth Services*, London: DfES.

Foot, P. (2002) *Moral Dilemmas*, Oxford: Oxford University Press.

Freidson, E. (2001) *Professionalism: The Third Logic*, Cambridge: Polity Press.

Gilligan, C. (1982) *In a Different Voice: Psychological Theory and Women's Development*, Cambridge, MA: Harvard University Press.

Held, V. (2006) *The Ethics of Care: Personal, Political, and Global*, Oxford: Oxford University Press.

Hursthouse, R. (1997) 'Virtue theory and abortion', in D. Statman (ed.) *Virtue Ethics: A Critical Reader*, Edinburgh: Edinburgh University Press.

Hursthouse, R. (1999) *On Virtue Ethics*, Oxford: Oxford University Press.

Jeffs, T. (1979) *Young People and the Youth Service*, London: Routledge & Kegan Paul.

Jeffs, T. and Smith, M. (2008) 'Valuing youth work', *Youth and Policy*, 100: 277–302.

Kant, I. (1785/1964) *Groundwork of the Metaphysics of Morals*, trans. H. Paton, New York: Harper & Row.

Koehn, D. (1994) *The Ground of Professional Ethics*, London: Routledge.

Kuhse, H. (1997) *Caring: Nurses, Women and Ethics*, Oxford: Blackwell.

Lifelong Learning UK (LLUK) (2008) *National Occupational Standards for Youth Work*, http://www.lluk.org (accessed September 2009).

MacIntyre, A. (1985) *After Virtue: A Study in Moral Theory*, 2nd edn, London: Duckworth.

Mendus, S. (1993) 'Different voices, still lives: problems in the ethics of care', *Journal of Applied Philosophy*, 10: 17–27.

Mill, J.S. (1863/1972) 'Utilitarianism', in *Utilitarianism, On Liberty, and Considerations on Representative Government*, London: Dent.

National Youth Agency (NYA) (2000) *Ethical Conduct in Youth Work: A Statement of Values and Principles from the National Youth Agency*, Leicester: The National Youth Agency.

Noddings, N. (1984) *Caring: A Feminine Approach to Ethics and Moral Education*, Berkeley and Los Angeles: University of California Press.

Noddings, N. (2002) *Starting at Home: Caring and Social Policy*, Berkeley and Los Angeles: University of California Press.

Oakley, J. and Cocking, D. (2001) *Virtue Ethics and Professional Roles*, Cambridge: Cambridge University Press.

Osborne, T. (1998) 'Constructionism, authority and the ethical life', in I. Velody and R. Williams (eds) *The Politics of Constuctionism*, London: Sage.

Payne, M. (2009) 'Modern youth work: purity or common cause', in J. Hine and J. Wood (eds) *Working with Young People*, London: Sage.

Quality Assurance Agency (QAA) (2009) *Subject Benchmark Statement: Youth and Community Work*, Gloucester: Quality Assurance Agency for Higher Education.

Schön, D. (1991) *The Reflective Practitioner: How Professionals Think in Action*, paperback edn, Aldershot: Avebury/Ashgate.

Siegrist, H. (1994) 'The professions, state and government in theory and history', in T. Becher (ed.) *Governments and Professional Education*, Buckingham: SRHE and Open University Press.

Slote, M. (2007) *The Ethics of Care and Empathy*, London: Routledge.

Spence, J., Devanny, C. and Noonan, K. (2007) *Youth Work: Voices of Practice*, Leicester: The National Youth Agency.

Statman, D. (1997) 'Introduction to virtue ethics', in D. Statman (ed.) *Virtue Ethics: A Critical Reader*, Edinburgh: Edinburgh University Press.

Swanton, C. (2003) *Virtue Ethics: A Pluralistic View*, Oxford: Oxford University Press.

Taylor, T. (2009) 'In defence of youth work', http://indefenceofyouthwork.wordpress.com/tag/youth-work (accessed July 2009).

Tronto, J. (1993) *Moral Boundaries: A Political Argument for an Ethic of Care*, London: Routledge.

Tucker, S. (2004) 'Youth working: professional identities given, received or contested?', in J. Roche, S. Tucker, R. Thomson and R. Flynn (eds) *Youth in Society*, 2nd edn, London: Open University Press/Sage.

Van Hooft, S. (2006) *Understanding Virtue Ethics*, Chesham: Acumen.

Verschelden, G., Coussée, F., Van De Walle, T. and Williamson, H. (2009) 'The history of youth work in Europe and its relevance for today's youth work policy, report from workshop, Blankenberge, Belgium, May 2008', http://youth-partnership.coe.int/youth-partnership/documents/EKCYP/Youth_Policy/docs/History/Research/Relevance_history.pdf (accessed July 2009).

Weber, M. (1978) *Economy and Society*, Berkeley: University of California Press.

Wittgenstein, L. (1972) *Philosophical Investigations*, trans. G.E.M. Anscombe, 3rd edn, Oxford: Blackwell.

<table>
<tr><td>

2

</td><td>

Working in welfare

</td></tr>
</table>

Youth policy's contradictions and dilemmas

Phil Mizen

Introduction

As human beings we live in societies whose structures and cultures seem to confront us as alien forces beyond our control, ways of living into which we involuntarily enter and whose presence is felt in terms of a powerful, sometimes determining, presence over the conduct of our lives. Yet as human beings we are also aware of our own powers to determine future courses of action. As active agents in possession of what sociologists may refer to as a uniquely reflexive quality, we hold understandings of how we exist in relation to the social contexts in and through which we live, and how these forces exert an influence over our preferred ways of living and working (Archer 2005). It is from this reflexive character, this essential and universal condition of human existence, that the powers of structural and cultural forces are mediated by us as human subjects. When faced with social contexts that appear to stand in our way or which we are not readily inclined to follow, it is from our reflexivity that we go about the redefinition of our ongoing concerns, draw upon those resources over which we can exercise some command, formulate new ways of working, and resist or cooperate with whatever it is that seems to impede our sense of what is right and proper.

This much is all too familiar for many welfare workers, even if it is more likely a consequence of their everyday experiences than engagement with the works of the most sophisticated sociologists. To work in welfare is to understand that the real and tangible differences that the welfare state can make to the lives of those tainted by circumstance, neglect or indifference are ones that often come to us in ways that remain unsatisfying or that seem to penalise. It is a longstanding and often articulated acknowledgement that the very real benefits which individuals derive from the welfare state may require its users (and workers) to subject themselves to varying degrees of supervision and control in ways that may bring the very idea of welfare into question. To respond to individuals on the basis of their need rather than their ability to pay and to activate the resources, time, knowledge or expertise that may enable someone to live a fuller life than may otherwise have been the case is knowingly to do so on terms not always of one's choosing.

It is knowledge of these terms of action that is the primary focus of this chapter. In considering the contradictions and dilemmas faced by youth workers it is necessary to know the context within which these are shaped and to understand the outcomes and implications of youth policy. In the following section, therefore, the particular relationship between young people and the state will be discussed, since it is from the administrative and policy functions of the state that young people's lives take much of their shape and substance. Following this, the next section will consider how this relationship between the state, youth policy and young people has changed in recent times and how with it there have been significant modifications to the terms upon which young people have been integrated into society. This will then be followed by an examination of the relationship between young people, and the principles, practices and outcomes of recent youth policy, focusing on the period from 1997 when 'New Labour' came to power in Britain. The next section begins to tease out some of the dilemmas that the current British government's youth policy poses at the time of writing (2009) for those seeking constructive and mutually productive working relationships with young people.

The state of youth

'Hard-headed analysis of policy has never before been more necessary', writes Bernard Davies (2006: 12); 'indeed, it has to remain a first tool of practice'. Elsewhere, I have written about the importance of state policy to youth and of how youth policy has been engulfed in successive crises (Mizen 2004). By this, I mean that much of what we have come to understand as youth is a consequence of the organisation of the state and especially of the forms of social administration that the state projects onto the lives of the young. Detached long ago from its basis in human physiology, youth has been defined more and more in terms of the political imperatives faced by governments as they have gone about the management of economic and social life, and the struggles over the distribution of resources that this involves. Key elements of this have included the institutionalisation of young people's dependence upon their families, the generalisation of compulsory education, the removal of children from the labour market, and a legal and moral framework to regulate marriage and sexual conduct. These changes to the parameters of young people's lives have been accompanied by significant adjustments to the fabric. In their dealings with young people, governments have sought to foster certain models of family conduct, educate young people in particular mores and values, shape the nature of youth's involvement in work, commerce and leisure, and encourage certain relationships among young people, the criminal justice system and the public systems of welfare support.

In thinking about youth in terms of the state and youth policy, two further matters are significant. First, in its dealings with young people, age has become an important means of social organisation. It is by reference to their chronological age, rather than individual needs or consideration of inequalities of class, gender or ethnicity, that the administrative apparatus of the state relates primarily to youth. Young people are especially aware of what this means in practice, as it is on the basis of age that they are separated from adults and from one another, and it is through age that they acquire important rights and responsibilities.[1] As anyone who works with the young quickly learns, this produces a keen sense of the arbitrariness of state power and young people well know how considerations of age are incapable of discerning an individual's capacity for action or of weighing up their needs. Young people are also among the first to point to the contradictory positions that age assigns to them. It can be a source of considerable frustration for young people in Britain to know that one can get married but not purchase an alcoholic drink to celebrate, or that liability for tax comes with no say in the election of governments responsible for spending this money.

Second, by considering youth in terms of age and state policy, we can also begin to understand better the terms of young people's integration into society. In relating to young people on the basis of chronological age, state policy attributes to youth a common quality as young people are organised into similar positions *vis-à-vis* the key social institutions and practices of the law, economy and democratic practice. Of course, this universal status serves a clear ideological function in its denial of the often wide social divisions between young people and the oppressions that usually flow from these divisions (Cohen 1997). Yet this administratively constituted youthful equivalence does have a substantive existence in its creation of common ways of living as young people that leave untouched more enduring sources of exploitation and division. For instance, it really is the case that *all* young people under a certain age must undergo education, but their common status as students denies the capacity of a small number of families to activate the economic and cultural resources to hand and that are usually necessary to secure educational (and thus social) advantage. My point is that in dealing with young people according to equivalence of age, youth policy works to reproduce important sources of social power and economic disadvantage. In relating to young people on the basis of age, this point of contact also provides the means to integrate young people into ways of living that are defined by the broader political configuration of social life.

The changing state of youth

One way of understanding how youth policy works to integrate young people into society, and how this has changed in recent years, is to think in terms of Keynesianism and monetarism/neo-liberalism. These terms are more familiar to economists than to youth workers, but they have value as ways of appreciating the state's contrasting attempts to organise social life in the second half of the twentieth century (LEWRG 1980). Keynesianism, characteristic of the years after World War Two, expresses a more inclusive form of state activity, one in which the state actively intervened to organise social life around a huge programme of concessions. The creation of the welfare state in particular took the influence of the state deep into the fabric of society so that its presence was felt not only in the public worlds of schooling and work, but also in the organisation of the family and in some of the most intimate aspects of personal life. With this extension of the state's reach and influence came important changes to its conduct, as considerations of individual need mitigated and displaced those of profitability, cost and market efficiency. Rather than relying on the market to meet the needs and aspirations of individuals and their families, the state actively intervened to create more conciliatory and inclusive forms of social organisation. The clearest expression of this was the universalism of the welfare state and its commitment to meet the needs of all outside of their ability to pay or the power they could command in the market.

This inclusive approach to the management of social relations was never sufficient to bring relief from the degradations of work or the privations of poverty, and public services remained inadequate and intrusive. Nevertheless, the concessions embodied in the Keynesian welfare state were real enough and the young were among its major beneficiaries. Many more teenagers, for instance, were removed from the labour market to an expanded education system that eschewed selection and proclaimed a more comprehensive ethos. Governments of both major political parties in Britain pledged themselves to manage the economy in ways that would guarantee jobs for all school leavers and young people enjoyed new forms of protection at work. The young also benefited from the extension of their participation in civil society through their inclusion in an expanded framework of civil, legal and political rights. Considerations of young people's needs as well as their deeds became a requirement of the administration of youth offending, while for a moment its decriminalisation became a real possibility (Newburn 1997). To administer to these changes the class of 'youth professionals' was greatly expanded. In the revamped schools and classrooms, newly created social services and children's departments, in the expanded careers, probation and youth services, professionals schooled in the latest theory and practice could bring their technical expertise to bear on the problems faced by those young people left behind by the pace of postwar change (Davies 1986).

As we all now know, boom turned quickly to bust, and what appeared as one of the benefits of this inclusive approach emerged as its greatest liability. In intervening directly in social relations, the state took on responsibility for the outcomes, and when times were good governments were quick to claim the credit. However, in the context of the failure of education to lead to jobs, rising youth unemployment, stagnating wages, deteriorating public services and the continuing rise in crime and disorder, by the 1970s the interventionist state also risked taking much of the blame for failure. It is in this context that a new form of politics gained ascendancy in which blame for the crisis was redirected away from the longer-term problems of British capitalism and laid firmly at the feet of the inclusive state. Arbitrary promises, unaccountable politicians and self-serving welfare bureaucrats, it was argued, had not only squandered valuable resources but had paradoxically created a demoralised and indolent youth underclass, undermined the work ethic and eroded the respect and deference that the young had traditionally held out to their elders and betters (Marsland 1996; Murray 1992; cf. Macdonald and Marsh 2005).

Criticisms such as these drew their force from changes already underway in how the state was seeking to organise social life and from its redrawing of its relationship with society and young people. In opposition to the interventionism and inclusivity of the Keynesian welfare state, neo-liberal and monetarist arguments expressed a much more exclusive approach to the management of social relations (Byrne 2005). This rejected earlier commitments to use state power to bring prosperity and welfare to *all*, and removed concession and conciliation as its *modus operandi*. Popular aspirations for rising living standards, jobs and improved welfare services could be returned to what the market was prepared to offer, and money took greater prominence as a way of organising social life. Considerations of cost rather than the services that people really needed were brought to the fore as cash limits were imposed upon the planning and delivery of public services and public expenditure was curbed. For the few commanding a significant income or in possession of considerable personal wealth, the turn to money presaged a remarkable improvement in standards of living. For those on the lowest incomes, the promise that this wealth would trickle down was never more than a hollow one.

With the rise of neo-liberalism, both the character and content of youth was subject to systematic restructuring. The inclusive strategy, it was claimed, had created a generation of young people lacking the work ethic and devoid of moral purpose: the muggers and hedonists, the work-shy and scroungers, the incivility and aimlessness of youth that so often filled the headlines. If being young had been elevated into a relatively good 'thing' to be under the inclusive strategy, and if being young meant a new inclusivity and significant additional public support, all this now needed sweeping away. The restructuring programme that emerged was both extensive in ambition and increasingly methodical in practice. Among its most prominent examples were the redesignation of education according to the 'needs' of employers, greater competitive pressures and a drastic erosion of funding. Governments also renounced earlier commitments to provide jobs for all with calls for aspirations to be brought more in line with what the market was prepared to offer. Young people's entitlements to welfare benefits were progressively withdrawn and the conditions of access to what remained made more selective. Any further moves towards the more humane treatment of young offenders were loudly condemned, while individual culpability and punishment were noisily reasserted.

Hard labour?

The history of youth policy tells us that the neo-liberal/monetarist strategy was even less successful than what it replaced (Mizen 2004), and it was from growing popular disillusionment that a Labour government was returned to power. Making much of these palpable failures, 'New Labour' came to power advocating a 'modernising agenda' that possessed a distinctively youthful theme. A decade after Bernard Davies (1986) first advanced the idea that the Thatcher governments were constructing a centrally controlled youth policy running counter to the pluralism and openness of what had gone before, there appeared something both paradoxical and disquieting about a Labour government championing a nationally coordinated policy framework for youth.

This said, New Labour's commitment to tackling the dreadful levels of 'social exclusion' experienced by young people during the monetarist/neo-liberal years has tempered anxieties (Coles 2000). Like all Labour governments before it, New Labour stood committed to social justice and welfare for all, and firmly rejected the neo-liberal confidence in unfettered market forces. And yet, as familiar as these aspirations are to Labour traditions, they nevertheless stand as part of a programme whose 'newness' is better understood by reference to the limits of the policy instruments deployed to realise them. Gone was any enduring commitment to the inclusiveness of the post-1945 settlement, and to use state power actively to manage market forces, regulate incomes or redistribute wealth. Missing too was the belief in the need to modify the structural inequalities and social divisions upon which the expansion of markets depend. Such goals and beliefs, indeed, are now anathema.

What is advocated in its place is 'the social investment state' (Giddens 1998: 117), where the state assumes the role of enabler and increased public investment is justified only in terms of its role in promoting market efficiency. We could perhaps better describe New Labour's attempt to reconcile a more prominent role for market forces with a renewal of the importance of social justice as one of 'progressive competitiveness', against the 'austere competitiveness' of the neo-liberal/monetarist years (Coates 2000). Significant increases in public expenditure and an expansion of the state's direct influence in social life are justified in terms of encouraging more efficient market relations as the means of organising social life, rather than their displacement or modification. This is especially true for education and training since, by investing in youth labour, in 'human capital', economic growth may be combined with greater welfare. By improving the supply of skilled and qualified young workers, on the one hand, the claim is that the United Kingdom will become more attractive to international investors which will, in turn, feed through into the creation of jobs. On the other hand, by providing more training and qualifications, young people can be made more 'employable', thus tackling the root cause of their 'social exclusion'. Individual young people will feel the benefits as skills and qualifications feed into access to jobs, more stable employment and higher earnings. In addition, the rewards to families and communities will be equally visible through improvements to social cohesion, as increased participation in education, training and work will remove the potential threat posed by large numbers of young people with empty time on their hands and nothing to do (Levitas 2005).

The commitment to social justice and the availability of new resources are clearly a welcome development, but the significant extension of compulsion that comes with them constitutes new concerns and dilemmas. Coercion is a necessary part of New Labour's youth policy because if the interests of the nation, communities and individuals are held to rely on greater social investment, the young must be obliged to conform. We witness this across the range of youth policy, in the crackdown on truancy and non-attendance at schools undergoing 'modernisation' through public–private rebuilding programmes, privatised academies and increased staffing levels; a punitive sanctions regime brought to bear on refusals to address 'employability' by enrolling on training programmes or by seeking advice from personal counsellors; or in the threats to liberty and well-being for those who decline to 'help themselves' on treatment programmes or new regimes of behavioural therapy. Most conspicuous of all is the prefacing of the pledge to get 'tough on the causes of crime' with the determination to be tough with young offenders (Smith 2005). With the failure of young people to embrace the new opportunities to remake themselves as 'responsible' citizens comes the criminalisation of their incivility and raucous behaviour, and the more conspicuous separation and exclusion of those who transgress the criminal law (Young 1999).

It also needs stating that for all this new investment, most of the 'solutions' offered by New Labour's marketisation of youth and youth policy are far from attractive, and this is another reason for youth policy's coercive edge. It is certainly the case that the official record of youth unemployment declined markedly under New Labour, but alongside the much-celebrated expansion of 'graduate jobs', those offering relatively high-skilled high-paid employment, the presence of low-skilled, low-waged and insecure working among the young has been further institutionalised (Byrne 2005). With poor-quality and precarious work still a reality for even greater numbers of school leavers, it comes as little surprise that the intensification and extension of education has further deepened young people's concerns over the value of qualifications or, in many instances, of the role of schooling per se (Macdonald and Marsh 2005). New training schemes, counselling and assessment programmes have done little to disturb the ambivalence that young people have long held for such measures (Mizen 2003). New resources, individually tailored plans, counselling or the introduction of information technology cannot hide from the young the role of these measures in hardening the degradation of their labour (Carpenter and Speeden 2007).

Some may perhaps take comfort from the fact that young people are not so easily fooled, but the prospects of avoidance and non-participation can be equally harmful. Whatever our own predilections as far as youth policy is concerned, it is nevertheless the case that large numbers of young people continue to confront New Labour's 'modernisation' programme by refusing to participate or by leaving their programmes early. A characteristic feature of the past 20 years has been the emergence of a new category designated 'Status Zero', the almost one million young people under the age of 18 who are 'NEETS', that is, not in employment, education or training schemes (Carpenter and Freda 2007). 'Making work pay' through the grudging inclusion of young people within the National Minimum Wage has also failed to make much headway against 30 years of declining youth wages and gross inequalities between what young people and their parents are paid. In addition, for those communities most affected by the decline in real wages, whose young people have had their benefits cut or disallowed and who are experiencing the worst effects of increases in child poverty and unprecedented inequalities of income and wealth, insult is added to injury by the attention they are given by the police and the youth justice system.

Ethics in an age of progressive competitiveness

Contradictions such as the ones I describe seem to pose perennial problems for many welfare workers. Today, as before, it is still the case 'that the welfare state gives us some of the things we need, gives us "benefits", but it does so in a certain way, in a way that puts us down or oppresses us' (LEWRG 1980: 53). Yet as both the state and its relationship to society have been restructured, and as this restructuring has brought about profound changes to young people's lives, these contradictions generate new dilemmas. For those who encounter these as they go about their work or who witness their embodiment in young people's daily lives, the advantages that youth policy undoubtedly offers come with new dilemmas. In activating those resources and sources of assistance that can and do make a demonstrable difference to the lives of young people, there is the real risk that the costs of their already austere predicament are further multiplied as, working in what are perceived to be their 'best interests', young people are cajoled into situations or relationships whose overall benefits are hazy or difficult to gauge.

For youth work these dilemmas are especially poignant because they go to the heart of some of its most cherished ideals. Compromise, concession and the blending of the state's welfare and coercive dimensions into mutually productive relationships have always been necessary features of modern youth work. We see these features in how the advantages that accrued to youth work, as it professionalised from its origins in the paternalism of the nineteenth century remoralisation and child-saving movements, came with pressure to contain the costs of postwar reconstruction and foster exclusive notions of citizenship (Davies 1986; France and Wiles 1997). They appear again in the tensions between the unique freedoms of detached youth work and demands to use these spaces to contain young people's striking use of leisure time. In both cases, however, the costs seemed justifiable in terms of the perceived outcomes. Tolerance of an institutionalised permissiveness encouraged and supported voluntary and non-coercive forms of association, while the absence of either a clearly defined curriculum or prescriptive pedagogy proved an important counterpoint to a schooling that frequently alienated. Youth workers could point with considerable justification to professional relationships built upon trust and mutual respect, and within those spaces eked out through the structured ambiguity of much youth work practice, bold, experimental and sometimes radical innovations were possible (Jeffs 1997).

Even with the assault on the inclusiveness of the postwar period these dilemmas retained a considerable degree of clarity. The championing of free market ideology, financial restraint and law and order, and the hostility to welfare and social justice, indeed to the very idea of society itself, meant that at least one knew where one stood in the face of emerging youth policy. The inclusiveness of the Keynesian welfare state had represented a clear advance on both what had gone before and what was offered in its place and so, for all its limitations and intrusiveness, important elements of it were worth defending politically and in everyday practice. The assault on the welfare state simultaneously represented an attack on inclusivity and rationality, on the well-being of the young and on the potential to develop solutions to the needs of young people as they saw them. Life was often difficult, posts were axed, funding withdrawn and resources made available on a more conditional basis, but the threat this presented to the key tenets of youth-centred education and practice was explicit.

It is, to say the least, somewhat exasperating that matters have turned out to be much more complicated under New Labour. Its stated opposition to the 'austere competitiveness' of free market ideology, its respect for social justice and commitment to opportunity for all, the reinvigoration of the idea of society, all these offer tantalising opportunities to restate and then transcend those progressive forms of working much more attuned to the historical sensibilities of youth work and to the needs of young people. The reality, of course, has been somewhat different and, instead of seeking to reaffirm how damaging and inequitable markets are as a basis for organising social life, we have witnessed their marked consolidation alongside a strengthening of the means of surveillance and supervision necessary for their imposition. In many respects New Labour's enchantment with the market seems to have added a much more punitive thrust to youth policy than could have been imagined 30 years ago. It is indeed a possibility that only a Labour government could have achieved the support from trade unions, welfare workers, teachers, educationalists and youth professionals necessary to make real such a punitive regime.

Maintaining individual integrity and effective practice in the face of this is not easy. The pressures pushing down on those who work with young people are considerable, to which may be added a deepening of the suspicion of welfare professionals and an effacing of their ability to know their clients' needs and to formulate effective responses. With New Labour's 'modernisation' of the welfare state has come a further erosion of the autonomy of welfare workers in general and a particular deepening of distrust of youth workers: the subversives, fantasists, idealists. In place of nurturing professional expertise and encouraging public service, however flawed such concepts may have been, the 'new managerialism' (Clarke and Newman 1997) and its love of all things actuarial has redefined state and policy in terms of the management of risk as opposed to the careful and systematic investigation of young people's problems as a means to the development of rational solutions. Professional judgement has been subordinated to service provision visibly warped by risk assessments, target-driven outcomes and performance-related payment, and a necessarily more instrumental approach to service delivery. Elsewhere, the effects of privatisation and competitive tendering are becoming clearer. Practices influenced by open access and informal association are under threat from the demands to maximise participation and the realisation of predetermined outcomes.

It is not simply that these constraints run against the grain of youth work's youth-centred ethos. There is also the risk that youth workers will be drawn into creating new working relationships with young people in which the exercise of direction and control is a more explicit and routine part of their function. In defining provision in terms of preconceived outcomes there is a real potential for a deepening of antagonisms between what young people see as in their best interest and those defined by service providers. Contractual relations and public service agreements now stipulate in fine detail what is required and how this is to be achieved, and the staging of funding adds to the disciplining power of money. New resources have, of course, attracted new players into the sector and these are a potential source of reinvigoration. Much work continues to be guided by a firm commitment to putting young people's needs first, and ways of 'doing things' in sympathy with the interests of communities are still possible (Carpenter and Freda 2007). However, it is the case that the spaces in which this work can flourish are under considerable pressure as the freedom to determine agendas, tolerate diverse and uncertain outcomes, indeed to allow serendipity to thrive, are further compressed in favour of the targets and outcomes so central to New Labour's 'modernisation.

Conclusion

I began this chapter by stating one of the central problems of social existence: as human beings we are ultimately responsible for the formation and transformation of society, but are ourselves formed and transformed in this process of shaping. I began with this problem because its place in any discussion of ethics and the contradictions involved in youth policy and youth work are of more than abstract significance. As individuals we possess powers and properties that are very different from the structures and cultures within and through which we live, but our relationship to these is nevertheless one of interdependence. Unlike the objective power of structures and cultures to constrain or enable, to give us things that we need but in ways not of our choosing, as agents we possess the powers and properties to entertain meanings, to formulate choices and then to act upon these choices. It is important to remember this because neither youth workers and welfare professionals, nor those who are the object of their attention, are autonomous, rational choice individuals who respond to incentives and punishments (the 'carrot and sticks' of New Labour's youth policy) in ways that are causally predicted. As human beings we respond to those structures and ideas that confront us as subjects, as individuals with a reflexive capacity that allows us to develop projects in the face of what we encounter, to respond in unanticipated ways, to choose enthusiastically to offer cooperation or collaboration, to stay silent, say 'no' or resist.

How could such a humanistic reading play out when it comes to the ethics of contemporary youth policy? How can we as individuals and workers resolve the dilemmas faced each day in ways that are positive and constructive? These are questions not easily answered but, in revisiting his seminal work on *Threatening Youth*, Bernard Davies (2006) is unequivocal that complicity is not an option. When faced with youth policy's more clearly coercive elements he suggests three 'unfinished' possibilities upon which we can reflect as the basis for future action. We can use the considerable expertise and experience of youth workers to pressure government and policy-makers and, in the process, bring youth professionals together in campaigns, lobby groups, trade unions or professional organisations where we can also draw strength and purpose from our encounters with like-minded individuals. We can also look to the law as a means to protect children and young people's human rights in the face of policies that, for instance, unreasonably restrict their freedom of movement and association. Or we can adopt the 'principled pragmatism' of workers 'in and against the state' (LEWRG 1980). As individuals whose responsibility it is to design and implement the fine details of youth policy, we have the capacity and vision to influence practice, procedures and outcomes by way of small acts of resistance, modification and reconstruction. Being 'in and against', Davies concludes, 'is the best, and on the ground the only, form of manoeuvring available to workers and managers committed to the best young person-centred practice they can achieve in unsympathetic or even hostile environments' (2006: 13).

Questions for reflection and discussion

1 To what extent can contemporary 'youth policy' be described as consisting of mutually co-existing beneficial and coercive dimensions ('carrots and sticks') aimed at getting young people to behave in particular ways?

2 How desirable are such 'youth policies', both for young people and those professionals working with and for them?

3 In what ways can youth workers and other professionals working with young people go about reconciling the demands of 'youth policy' with the 'best interests' of young people?

Recommended reading

Levitas, R. (2005) *The Inclusive Society? Social Exclusion and New Labour*, 2nd edn, Basingstoke: Palgrave. A fine account of New Labour's approach to poverty and the poor, and its underlying philosophical and political principles. The book argues that in reclaiming questions of social justice and egalitarianism, New Labour redefined its aspirations to fairness and equality in ways that jettisoned much of its historical commitment to redistributive welfare. In its place, New Labour discourse increasingly emphasised the more efficient use of market forces as the primary source of individual welfare.

London Edinburgh Weekend Return Group (1980) *In and Against the State,* London: Pluto Press. Although perhaps somewhat dated, this book provided a timely critique of the social democratic welfare state and the dilemma it posed for progressive people working in the public/welfare sector. The book stresses the antagonistic position of welfare workers as they seek to utilise the enablements provided by the welfare state, while simultaneously having to deal with its coercive and disciplinary dimensions. Short, succinct and to the point, it is still well worth reading for welfare workers today.

Mizen, P. (2004) *The Changing State of Youth*, Basingstoke: Palgrave. A detailed account of 'youth policy' from the crisis of the social democratic welfare state of the 1970s through to the renewed commitment to young people's welfare espoused by the first Blair government. The book deals with a range of youth policies, including education, housing and youth justice and offending, but its principal focus is on work, unemployment and the training state.

Note

1 For an extensive chronology of youth policy see 'Youth Policy in the UK: A Chronological Map', www.keele.ac.uk/depts/so/youthchron/

References

Archer, M.S. (2005) *Making Our Way Through the World: Human Reflexivity and Social Mobility*, Cambridge: Cambridge University Press.

Byrne, D. (2005) *Social Exclusion*, 2nd edn, Maidenhead: Open University Press.

Carpenter, M. and Freda, B. (2007) 'Youth discrimination and labour market access: from transitions to capabilities', in M. Carpenter, B. Freda and S. Speeden (eds) *Beyond the Workfare State: Labour Markets, Equality and Human Rights*, Bristol: Policy Press.

Carpenter, M. and Speeden, S. (2007) 'Origins and effects of New Labour's workfare state: modernisation or variation on old themes?', in M. Carpenter, B. Freda and S. Speeden (eds) *Beyond the Workfare State: Labour Markets, Equality and Human Rights*, Bristol: Policy Press.

Clarke, J. and Newman, J. (1997) *The Managerial State: Power, Politics and Ideology in the Remaking of Welfare*, London: Sage.

Coates, D. (2000) *Models of Capitalism: Growth and Stagnation in the Modern Era*, Cambridge: Polity Press.

Cohen, P. (1997) *Rethinking the Youth Question*, Basingstoke: Macmillan.

Coles, B. (2000) *Joined-up Youth Research, Policy and Practice: A New Agenda for Change?*, Leicester: Youth Work Press.

Davies, B. (1986) *Threatening Youth*, Milton Keynes: Open University Press.

Davies, B. (2006) 'Threatening youth revisited: youth policies under New Labour', *The Encyclopaedia of Informal Education*, www.infed.org/archives/bernard_davies/revisiting_threatening_youth.htm (accessed 20 August 2006).

France, A. and Wiles, P. (1997) 'Dangerous fortunes: social exclusion and youth work in late modernity', *Social Policy and Administration*. 31: 59–78.

Giddens, A. (1998) *The Third Way*, Cambridge: Cambridge University Press.

Jeffs, T. (1997) 'Youth work and the "underclass" theory', in R. Macdonald (ed.) *Youth, The 'Underclass' and Social Exclusion*, London: Routledge.

Levitas, R. (2005) *The Inclusive Society? Social Exclusion and New Labour*, 2nd edn, Basingstoke: Palgrave.

London Edinburgh Weekend Return Group (LEWG) (1980) *In and Against the State*, London: Pluto Press.

Macdonald. R. and Marsh, J. (2005) *Disconnected Youth? Growing Up in Britain's Poor Neighbourhoods*, Basingstoke: Palgrave Macmillan.

Marsland, D. (1996) *Welfare or Welfare State?*, Basingstoke: Macmillan.

Mizen, P. (2003) 'The best days of your life? Youth, policy and Blair's New Labour', *Critical Social Policy*, 23: 453–476.

Mizen, P. (2004) *The Changing State of Youth*, Basingstoke: Palgrave Macmillan.

Murray, C. (1992) *The Underclass in Britain,* London: Institute for Economic Affairs.

Newburn, T. (1997) 'Youth, crime and justice', in M. Maguire, R. Morgan and R. Reiner (eds) *The Oxford Handbook of Criminology,* Oxford: Oxford University Press.

Smith, R. (2005) 'Actuarialism and early intervention in contemporary youth justice', in B. Goldson and J. Muncie (eds) *Youth Crime and Justice*, London: Sage.

Young, J. (1999) *The Exclusive Society*, London: Sage.

3 Ethics, collaboration and the organisational context of youth work

Kenneth McCulloch and Lyn Tett

Introduction

This chapter draws on a theoretical framework for mapping ethical climates in organisations and on research on primary and secondary schools as contexts for inter-professional collaboration, to explore how different aspects of context may interact and influence the ways in which ethical issues are understood and acted upon. We argue that analysis of professionalism and of the organisational context of youth work are central to our understandings of, and responses to, ethical problems.

We examine the ways in which workers, managers and organisations interact to facilitate or impede ethical practice in youth work. The organisations that employ youth workers are themselves diverse, and the chapter uses the concept of 'climates' for ethical decision-making to explore these differences. Because youth workers are increasingly required to work in organisational contexts characterised by the collaboration of different kinds of professional practitioners (for example, teachers, social workers and health professionals) particular attention is given to the significance of collaboration across professional boundaries and between organisations. Each of these professional communities has particular traditions and perspectives on ethical practice, and in the section on collaboration we explore how youth workers' understanding of their own role, and the expectations others have of them, will frame the context within which problems are both set and solved.

Professionalism and accountability

Professional and *professionalism* are not simply neutral, descriptive terms but are value laden and strongly contested. Wilding's (1982) critique represents professions as controlling and legitimising structures, operating in the interests of members of the particular professional group. Alternatively, professionalism may be understood as representing 'competence and [a] collective service ideal' (Airaksinen 1994: 1). We follow Freidson (1986) in using the term 'professionalism' to refer to a set of occupational practices and by extension attitudes and beliefs. These form the common bond for a community of practitioners who also share a body of knowledge. However, neither the particular knowledge, nor the practices that spring from that knowledge, is fixed and unchanging. Recognition of the dynamic nature of the relationship between these elements is vital to an understanding of professionalism in youth work.

As Holdsworth (1994: 43) points out, 'the professional has knowledge which other people do not have' and so is accountable for the ways in which such knowledge is used. Moreover, acting as a professional requires an attitude and approach that has to incorporate critical thinking and reflective practice. We believe that the diversity of youth work practice, which includes the volunteer giving a few hours to youth work as well as those who make it a full-time vocation, is encompassed in such a definition. The idea of professional*ism* follows from that, as a set of attitudes and practices to which any youth worker may aspire, whatever their level of training and qualifications.

Accountability necessarily has to take account of the guiding principles of a profession and involves judgement in synthesising conflicting objectives and values. However, a key characteristic of accountability is the expectation from both service users and the public at large that 'people must explain themselves to each other' (Holdsworth 1994: 44). This involves accepting responsibility for providing the fullest and most open account of our activities so that others may make judgements about our actions. Accountability also involves considering to whom workers are answerable – the profession, the organisation, the service users/young people or their own conscience. Conflicting accountabilities often present workers with their most acute dilemmas about what constitutes ethical practice.

By ethical practice we mean action that leads to human well-being from a perspective that values dispositions to truthfulness and justice. As Smith (1994: 76) points out, ethical practice 'entails an orientation to "good" or "right" rather than "correct" action . . . and allows people to break a rule or convention if they judge that to follow it would not promote "the good"'. At the heart of such practice is the principle of respect for persons, which 'relates to other principles such as autonomy, non maleficence, beneficence, equity and justice' (Henry 1994: 146).

The relationship between professionalism and professional values on the one hand, and organisational imperatives and accountability to an employer on the other, is a central issue for youth workers. The report of the Cullen Inquiry (Scottish Office 1996) led to increasing attention being paid to who may claim the label of 'youth worker' in Scotland, and more recently movements towards formal registration and the establishment of occupational standards have emerged. The central concerns here are with how professionalism is conceived, and how differing organisational contexts for youth work can both influence the ways in which professionalism is understood and constrain or direct workers' beliefs and activities.

Youth workers historically had considerably greater autonomy in determining their work priorities than is common in other professions such as teaching and social work. However, this has also meant that the underpinning beliefs, values and norms about what is appropriate practice may not be subject to much day-to-day challenge. Where choices are made in a context where ends are not determinate and value conflicts exist about both ends and means, judgement is crucial and will be guided by each individual's 'theory in use' (Argyris and Schön 1974). If youth workers are to explore their experiences and ethical accountability, they therefore need to become aware of what the prevailing norms and 'common-sense' views implicit in their practice are regarding practising what is preached. As Henry (1994: 145) points out:

> professional accountability is central to the setting of standards and norms, and persons within the organisation are responsible for planning and managing the quality and delivery of the service, both individually and collectively. From a professional perspective there is personal and collective accountability for establishing and maintaining the standards of practice.

Another important consideration is the way in which workers are held to be accountable to their organisations for the work that they do. Different conceptions of purpose are likely to result in different emphases on what is measured, whether these are processes, outputs or inputs. For example, a small local youth club would be likely to rate its financial independence and ability to recruit voluntary leaders as key measures of success, while a large national voluntary organisation like Barnardos or Save the Children might place emphasis on the extent to which vulnerable young people were enabled to remain in their own locality rather than being taken into some kind of residential care. In local authority settings, youth workers' concerns for acting in what they regard as the interests of the young people might conflict with a council's policy. This also illustrates how concern for ethical practice can lead to conflicts that result in people breaking rules that are seen to be concerned with 'correct' rather than 'right' action. Issues of professionalism and accountability are enacted, however, in particular organisational contexts, so we now turn to the relationship between organisational context and professional cultures.

The organisational context: four 'climates' of ethical practice

In general our focus is more on culture and processes than on structural factors such as organisational systems. The notion of organisational culture is somewhat problematic but, for our purposes, we will use the following definition:

> Organisational culture is defined here as a patterned system of perceptions, meanings and beliefs about the organisation which facilitates sense-making amongst a group of people sharing common experiences and guides individual behaviour at work.
>
> (Bloor and Dawson 1994: 276)

These authors offer a useful model for the interpretation of professional cultures and subcultures in their organisational context, emphasising the importance of 'patterns of signification, legitimation and domination' (Giddens, cited in Bloor and Dawson 1994: 278). The example of medical dominance over partner professions such as physiotherapy and social work offers a parallel with both collaboration and with the problem of inter-professional relations within, for example, a local authority. Similarly, youth workers practising in a context where there is a statutory social work dimension to the relationship with young people may find their concerns and priorities subjugated to those of their social work colleagues.

Millar (1995) has argued that many youth services operate in a 'person' culture, in which the needs and desires of individuals within the organisation take precedence over the demands of the organisation itself, and this orientation can lead to an oppositional stance to authority. We would agree that the professional culture of youth work can lead to a view of management as inherently problematic since in many of its manifestations it will be seen as antithetical to the dominant value-base that defines youth workers' professionalism. Drawing on The National Youth Agency's (2004) statement on ethical conduct, Banks (2009: 51) outlines the principles underpinning youth work practice as: respect for young people as persons and as autonomous decision-makers; concern for young people's welfare and safety; commitment to social justice; and, finally, professional integrity. This may mean that activist youth workers may see managers as part of a structure of social authority that is oppressing the very people for whom they are seeking to establish equality of opportunity (Case study 9.2 (p. 148) illustrates this point).

Workers experience the organisations within which they function as influencing their activities in many different ways. Organisations may impose rules or rely on workers' judgements; they may encourage or stifle innovation at the grass roots; they control resources such as time, money or equipment. The smallest and largest organisations may behave in similar ways in this latter respect, even though the resource concerned might range from a five- or six-figure sum of money to control over the keys to the scout hut. Such tensions between organisational imperatives and the value positions that influence youth workers' purposes and behaviour lead us on to consider the concept of 'ethical climate' in organisations.

The concept of work climate is chosen to represent a sense of 'how it feels to work here' in terms of the range of conditions for professional practice that may be encountered by youth workers. Victor and Cullen (1988: 101) characterise work climate in the ethical sense as 'the prevailing perceptions of typical organisational practices and procedures that have ethical content'. From an organisational point of view this is represented as the way in which individuals perceive their activities and autonomy as being more or less *pre*scribed, *pro*scribed or requiring permission.

We have developed the typology represented as Figure 3.1, where our first key dimension (along the horizontal axis) is accountability and different understandings of the 'professional'. The second dimension (on the vertical axis) represents the ethical criterion manifest in the organisational priority given to right action or conversely to such criteria as public image. Like many such typologies it is somewhat simplified, since the dimensions proposed represent complex concepts, which are here reduced to bipolar constructs. It is also important to recognise the limits of such a theoretical model; the realities experienced by workers in their working lives will be more subtle and complex than can be fully explained by a conceptualisation of this kind.

We suggest that accountability may be conceived of in terms of control by the organisation or, by contrast, by reference to a professional ideal or ethic. This

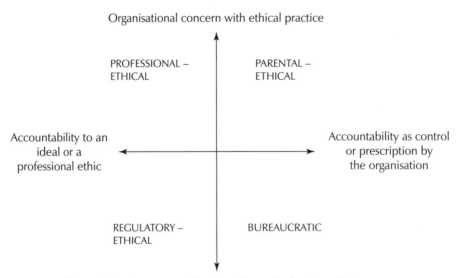

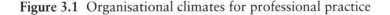

Figure 3.1 Organisational climates for professional practice

polarity provides one dimension of our framework (the horizontal axis in Figure 3.1) premised on competing representations of the professional – *the trained practitioner* and *reflective professional* ideals. The second dimension is represented as concern with organisational integrity and reputation versus concern with ethical practice or 'the good' (vertical axis). The two axes are not, however, of precisely equal significance. The accountability dimension is stronger simply because the effects of organisational priority on practice will tend to be less influential where practice ethics are derived from professionalism rather than from an organisational prescription. This framework enables us to conceptualise the climates of organisations in what we have chosen to describe as professional-ethical, regulatory-ethical, parental-ethical and bureaucratic approaches to ethical practice.

The notion of inter-organisational collaboration adds a further layer of complexity. We have not sought to represent this graphically, but it may be thought of as increasing the size or changing the shape of the space in this conceptual map that workers experience themselves occupying. We will now describe briefly each of the four quadrants of Figure 3.1 in turn.

Bureaucratic

Originally conceptualised as a way of describing an ideal form of organisation for complex tasks, the classical bureaucracy (Weber 1947) is characterised by well-defined lines of communication and accountability, clearly delineated job boundaries and distinct levels of authority to make decisions. The scope for autonomous action is limited, and professionalism therefore becomes problematic in the sense that the organisation's imperatives are ascribed a superordinate or at least equal standing with professional codes. Consideration of the occupations characterised by Etzioni (1969) as 'semi-professions', for example, social work and nursing, reveals activities which are characteristically quite highly supervised and more often than not operate within a framework of bureaucratic hierarchy such as a local government administration or a hospital.

In a local authority we may find that youth workers experience it as a constraining bureaucracy, concerned primarily to achieve corporate objectives and avoid criticism, and expecting professional staff to pursue the corporate purpose and to account for their actions within that framework. It may not, however, be the case that bureaucracy is entirely inimical to youth workers. One might argue that clear organisational guidance about what is and what is not desirable or permissible in practice may well help workers to clarify objectives, and to routinise a range of decisions that would otherwise take up resources of time and energy. Conversely, an organisational context that tends to deny or stifle professional autonomy may be more likely to lead to atrophy of the ethical sense and to a loss of workers' capacity to make their own professional judgements and to have confidence in their capacity to do so.

There may be a tendency for larger, more diversified organisations to be less respectful of the professional autonomy to which youth workers might believe themselves entitled. In a collaborative environment, staff will not necessarily be managed and supervised by professional peers and the autonomy of workers to follow their own judgements, or even to adopt a distinctive stance on an issue such as work with young people on sexuality issues, is severely constrained. By contrast, in a more peer-led community, innovation is encouraged and the taking of risks is, within limits, supported rather than criticised, even when the outcomes are less than ideal.

Parental-ethical

This label emerged as an appropriate characterisation of an organisation concerned to do the right thing but reluctant to trust the worker to make independent decisions about what courses of action to follow. In transactional analysis terms (Berne 1964) it would be seen as a 'controlling parent', and the emphasis on accountability through control or prescription by the organisation makes the notion of professionalism problematic. Some degree of autonomy is an important dimension of professionalism, and it is therefore difficult to so characterise work in an organisation which functions in this way, even though such a culture may be found in many of the traditional professions.

It is not hard to find examples of settings where informal work with young people is conducted in such an atmosphere. Uniformed organisations with their quasi-military structures and symbols might be characterised in this way, emphasising quite specific schemes of work and a strong hierarchy. Similarly, many organisations of the small voluntary club type operate effectively under the control of one strong individual, or at most a very small group. There is nothing inherently problematic about such a climate. The critical tension in such a climate is likely to be between the dominant centre and potential alternative leadership. Alternative conceptions of purpose are effectively excluded unless control shifts from one dominant individual or group to a new centre of power.

Regulatory-ethical

Here, accountability is to an ideal or professional ethic. The worker's loyalty is at least as much to a wider community of practice and to those they serve, as it is to the employer. Scope for autonomy is acknowledged and treated as an entitlement, albeit constrained by the organisation's concern with its reputation or public image. Workers cannot be permitted to exercise their discretion in ways that might appear to threaten that image. The central difficulty for the worker in this climate is to maintain commitment to the idealised notions of professional practice while avoiding transgression of the organisation's imposed norms.

A regulatory-ethical climate is typical of the conditions under which many established professional groups operate. The moral authority of the professional community itself and an employing organisation carry about equal weight and would only rarely tend to exert conflicting influences. In a youth work context the particular character of an agency or organisation often largely determines ethical boundaries. For example, in a large national organisation with many staff and a range of activities, boundaries are set internally and are legitimated in part by the history and standing of the organisation. In a smaller independent project, by contrast, workers may see the main source of authority as lying outside the project itself, in the hands of funders. The mediation of this authority through the framework of an independent project creates a protective barrier, and provides the project and its workers with the standing of autonomous professionals. At the same time the constraint of 'funder acceptance' is rarely out of sight. Despite the ambiguities which are clearly present, workers may see such a climate as attractive; it would perhaps be evidenced by a moderate turnover of staff, clear commitments to ethical practice in openness to the critical questioning of decisions, proactive training and staff development policies and innovative practice.

Professional-ethical

The combination of an organisation concerned at a corporate level to act ethically, and of individuals' independent accountability to a professional ethic may seem to be an ideal to strive towards. In practice, however, a number of potential difficulties may appear. The requirement for fully conscious decision-making by 'autonomous professionals' creates a level of demand on the individual worker that may be difficult to sustain. Primary reference to a 'community of practice' (Wenger 1998) rather than to organisational rules or simply custom and practice as the source of support in ethical decision-making may leave the individual experiencing isolation, doubt and uncertainty as a consequence of any dilemma with an ethical dimension.

It seems unlikely that many youth workers will find themselves working in such a climate, although a lack of close scrutiny over practice and the isolation of individual workers sometimes create the impression that one is working in an 'ethical' climate when the reality is more appropriately understood as an ineffective bureaucracy. As a work climate it may also lack the focus for debate and the resolution of conflict, although it could be claimed that this kind of debate is simply transferred from the immediate surroundings of the organisation to some professional forum where issues are explored, disputes resolved and transgressors sanctioned. It is better in our view for the nature and purpose of practice to be the focus of regular scrutiny and discussion by one's peers, in the context of practice rather than outside it.

Any notion of a theoretical 'ideal' climate will vary according to, among other factors, the nature and purpose of the work. However, if pressed we would tend to concentrate on the stronger accountability axis and seek a position towards the idealised notion of accountability to a professional ethic rather than to organisational control. This is not, however, to suggest that other climates are unavoidably hostile. Climate as a metaphor allows us to anticipate that professionalism may be able to survive and even flourish in a range of situations. It is also important to recognise that a theoretical model of this kind will not offer a perfect fit with every real-life situation.

Collaboration

In this section we focus on situations in which youth workers work collaboratively with other professionals because issues around professionalism and accountability are most likely to arise in these contexts. Youth workers commonly find themselves working in inter-agency groups where they are collaborating, for example, with teachers in school-based programmes, with social workers in areas such as youth justice and welfare, and with health professions in health promotion and education. They also work inter-professionally within, for example, youth offending teams where different professionals based in the same teams and offices work together. All of these collaborations bring with them the potential for conflict and tension, in ethical and other domains, alongside their potential for productive outcomes.

This is partly because collaboration requires a change in approach that seeks to minimise differences in aims, culture and procedures between people that have different traditions of working. Milburn (1994) has suggested that much collaboration is 'phantom' because different workers and different organisations continue to work in parallel rather than by changing practices. 'True' collaboration would lead to 'collaborative advantage' (Huxham 1996, 2003) where something unusually creative is produced that is more than the sum of the contributing parts, and may lead to some benefit for wider society that is beyond the remit of any of the participating organisations themselves. However, misunderstandings, antagonism, differences in values and differential expectations from the host organisations in relation to the accountability and availability of staff can seriously affect collaborative work. Interestingly, it is often only in collaboration with other professions that youth workers may become aware of their underlying professional values when they find themselves challenged to justify particular ways of acting (see Banks 2009).

Collaboration between different organisations will almost always generate a complex web of conflicts about ends, means and values. At the simplest level staff and board members of an independent youth project may feel railroaded into taking particular action by the local council because it provides a large proportion of its income. From the perspective of the project staff and managers they are certainly not engaging in 'true' collaboration that would result in mutually agreed action. Similarly, volunteers may have very different views about the purposes of their club from paid staff and hence working together on a project that had shared aims and objectives can be problematic. Collaborative practice can also lead to many advantages for organisations such as the *more effective use of resources* and skills, enhanced creativity, improved services for young people and increased staff confidence. However, it takes time and effort and an awareness of the context to enable effective work to take place.

In order to illustrate how inter-agency and inter-professional collaborations impact upon youth workers we now turn to two research projects we conducted that focused on primary and secondary schools (McCulloch *et al.* 2004; Tett *et al.* 2001). In these projects youth workers employed by a variety of organisations, including small independent projects, national voluntary organisations and local authorities, collaborated with a range of other professionals including schoolteachers, social workers, nurses and the police in order to engage with young people who had been designated as 'at risk'.

In one collaborative project we examined, a council had contracted a small voluntary sector organisation to provide out-of-school activities for young people as part of an alternative curriculum for those who were regarded by the secondary school as exhibiting antisocial behaviour. The youth workers collaborated with the young people, the school's guidance and support teachers and the pupils' parents to develop a programme that was based on the young people's interests and strengths rather than a prescribed curriculum that they regarded as emphasising their deficits. In their interactions with the council the youth workers saw the ethos that the council operated within as largely reflecting a concern to achieve corporate objectives and avoid criticism where the staff were expected to pursue the council's purpose of minimising risk. They perceived the council as operating within a *bureaucratic climate* whereas in their own organisation they were much more used to being part of a peer-led community where they were encouraged to be innovative in responding to the ideas of the young people and received support in setting ambitious objectives even if they did not always achieve them. This conflict might have stifled their capacity to make their own professional judgements, but this dilemma was overcome by working on the one hand with the school staff, parents and young people in ways that accorded with their own ethos while, on the other, making sure that the objectives and outcomes of the project were reported using the guidelines that the council had provided. In this way they managed to work within a *regulatory-ethical climate* where the council provided the project and its workers with the standing of autonomous professionals who were free to work with young people in the ways they considered to be appropriate, but at the same time they operated under the constraints imposed by their funder in terms of meeting the council's predetermined outcomes.

Another example of collaboration took place in a school cluster comprising a secondary school and its feeder primary schools. This project had developed a structure where all referrals about 'at-risk' pupils were channelled through a single person who then convened a group of professionals and coordinated their responses so that the pupil and his or her carers had only one point of contact. In this example the one youth worker who was part of this team found himself operating within a *professional-ethical* climate. This was because he saw his accountability as being to the ethics of his professional community of practice (i.e. other youth workers) in the context of the inter-professional team where a range of professional codes were operating. This meant that the professional isolation he might otherwise have experienced was mitigated by discussion with his professional peers who were located outside of the collaboration. This was particularly important when an ethical dilemma, such as whether to give priority to young people's voice and participation in a situation where other professionals viewed this as a low priority, could be scrutinised and explored in discussion with his peers.

A final example from our research (McCulloch *et al.* 2004; Tett *et al.* 2001) arose when schools were seeking collaborating partners to work with in areas that they saw as beyond their own expertise, such as sexual health education. In this case youth workers appeared to be operating at times within a *parental-ethical* climate as the schools in which they worked exercised control over the content of the teaching and learning materials they were expected to use in their discussions with pupils. Thus, although the workers were using professional judgement in order to ensure that they respected and responded to the young people's views in the way in which they delivered their sessions, in other respects they had to follow the requirements of the school curriculum. The youth workers perceived the prescriptive curriculum as controlling in some respects, but by exerting some autonomy in their method of delivering the material they were able to exercise their professional judgement about how the young people might best be engaged and supported.

This example also demonstrates the power differentials that operate when different professions and/or agencies have divergent views about what collaboration means. For example, research has shown (e.g. Hatcher and Leblond 2001; Tett 2001) that from the perspective of schools effective collaboration stems from the capacity of other partners to add value to the schools' efforts in areas they regard as peripheral or difficult, such as sexual health education. Schools do not want to collaborate over 'core' activities such as the teaching of subject knowledge.

As may be seen from the above examples, collaborative partnerships are generally characterised by plural sets of values linked to different forms of expertise (Wilson and Pirrie 2001). Conflict and tension are inevitably part of the collaborative process and partnerships may be seen as a threat rather than a benefit (see Hatcher and Leblond 2001). Different partners bring differential forms of power and some have greater control as a result. In collaborations concerned with young people we may variously find conditions where different professional groups are required by ethical and legal frameworks to approach individuals or groups of young people in different ways and with different purposes in mind. For example, social workers will be expected to prioritise child protection, police officers law enforcement, youth workers young people's voice and participation, and so on.

The deep-rooted cultural differences between professional groups, vested interests in maintaining organisational and departmental boundaries and statutory restrictions may undermine efforts to engage in partnership working. This means that an increase in joint working has to be facilitated if inter-organisational collaboration is to succeed. In our research local authorities that appointed people with particular responsibility for promoting this collaboration seemed to be the most successful (McCulloch and Tett 2008). We also found that youth workers were more likely to be committed to collaboration and to become 'boundary spanners' (Ranade and Hudson 2003: 46), enabling the concept of integrated provision to become embedded in people's thinking. Such individuals 'appear to develop more complex models of social problems, and broader, more inclusive solutions than the more restricted perspectives of any one profession or agency' (Ranade and Hudson 2003: 46).

Conclusion

While collaboration might seem to present a problem for youth workers who see their purpose as concerned with young people's voice, participation and citizenship, a more optimistic analysis is possible. In a social work context, Dabby *et al.* (2008) argue for a postmodernist conception of ethics, where ethics is seen as a collaborative, dialogical activity involving the legitimate participation and contributions of anyone with an interest in the particular practice setting. On this view, ethical decision-making is as much the business of the users of a service, and of the different professional groups that might be involved, as it is the business of a formal professional body in its ethical codes and their enforcement. Based on this analysis, collaboration offers potential for a more dynamic and flexible ethical climate characterised by mutually respectful exchanges among professional groups, clients and practitioners. Collaboration also involves crossing boundaries between different practices, and this exposes our experience to different forms of engagement, different professions with different definitions of what matters, and different repertoires and ethics. As Wenger argues (1998: 140), 'by creating a tension between experience and competence, crossing boundaries is a process by which learning is potentially enhanced [but also] potentially impaired'.

We have shown that individuals, managers and organisations interact to facilitate or impede ethical practice in youth work, but that individual workers have the ability to interpret their own organisational context and act to integrate professional and organisational imperatives. Workers have a sense of agency; a belief that they can act to change the world they inhabit and that they can make a difference. Individual conceptions of ethical practice that have been forged through professional training, discussions with fellow workers or shared commitments to a particular value-base will result in actions that may differ from those espoused by the organisation. For example, in terms of accountability there can be real disagreements about how and to whom services are responsive when disruptive young people are construed by some workers as needing support and by 'management' as spoiling the provision for the majority. What this chapter has sought to demonstrate is not that such disagreements are avoidable, but that placing the exploration and resolution of debate at the heart of our work is essential. Ignoring the diversity of views that arise from the interactions in and between individuals and their organisations will not avoid disputes but simply 'displace them into discontent' (Fairley and Paterson 1995: 34). Being aware of the differing conceptions of professionalism, accountability and organisational context that we have explored is more likely to result in uncomfortable dilemmas and contradictions for individuals but, nevertheless, the struggle to resolve these will lead to growth and development and a more ethically based practice.

Questions for reflection and discussion

1 How are decisions about how to deal with ethical dilemmas dealt with in your workplace or an organisation with which you are associated?

2 Where would you place this organisation on the 'ethical climates' diagram?

3 How has the need to collaborate with partners from different traditions and disciplines influenced your own or your colleagues' ethical decision-making?

Recommended reading

Chadwick, R. (ed.) (1994) *Ethics and the Professions*, Aldershot: Avebury. Explores a range of themes and concepts in relation to professional ethics, drawing on a wide range of cases and contexts.

Huxham, C. (ed.) (1996) *Creating Collaborative Advantage*, London: Sage. Develops theoretical frameworks for understanding the potential and limits of collaboration.

Riddell, S. and Tett, L. (eds) (2001) *Education, Social Justice and Inter-agency*

Working: Joined up or Fractured Policy?, London: Routledge. Interrogates the policy context of inter-agency working and partnerships in education, drawing on examples from UK and international contexts.

References

Airaksinen, T. (1994) 'Service and science in professional life', in R. Chadwick (ed.) *Ethics and the Professions*, Aldershot: Avebury Press.

Argyris, C. and Schön, D. (1974) *Theory in Practice: Increasing Professional Effectiveness*, San Francisco, CA: Jossey Bass.

Banks, S. (2009) 'Values and ethics in work with young people', in J. Wood. and J. Hine (eds), *Work With Young People: Developments in Theory, Policy and Practice,* London: Sage.

Berne, E. (1964) *Games People Play*, New York: Grove Press.

Bloor, G. and Dawson, P. (1994) 'Understanding professional culture in organisational context', *Organisation Studies*, 15: 275–295.

Dabby, M., Faisal, H., Holliman, D., Karliner, S., Pearl, D. and Silverman, B. (2008) 'Ethics as activity: building collaborative, expansive and just social work' *Journal of Social Work Values and Ethics*, 5. Available at www.socialworker.com/jswve/content/view/91/65/ (accessed 1 May 2009).

Etzioni, A. (1969) *The Semi-professions and their Organisation*, London: Collier Macmillan.

Fairley, J. and Paterson, L. (1995) 'Scottish education and the new managerialism', *Scottish Educational Review*, 27: 13–36.

Freidson, E. (1986) *Professional Powers: A Study of the Institutionalisation of Formal Knowledge*, Chicago, IL, and London: University of Chicago Press.

Hatcher, R. and Leblond, D. (2001) 'Education Action Zones and Zones d'Education Prioritaires', in S. Riddell and L. Tett (eds) *Education, Social Justice and Inter-agency Working: Joined Up or Fractured Policy?*, London: Routledge.

Henry, C. (1994) 'Professional behaviour and the organisation', in R. Chadwick (ed.) *Ethics and the Professions*, Aldershot: Avebury Press.

Holdsworth, D. (1994) 'Accountability: the obligation to lay oneself open to criticism', in R. Chadwick (ed.) *Ethics and the Professions*, Aldershot: Avebury Press.

Huxham, C. (ed.) (1996) *Creating Collaborative Advantage*, London: Sage.

Huxham, C. (2003) 'Seeking collaborative advantage: a themes-based theory', *Public Management Review,* 5: 401–423.

McCulloch, K and Tett, L. (2008) 'Integrated community schools and social inclusion (Scotland)', in M. Baginsky (ed.) *Safeguarding Children and Schools*, London: Jessica Kingsley.

McCulloch, K., Tett, L. and Crowther, J. (2004) 'New community schools in Scotland: issues for inter-professional collaboration', *Scottish Educational Review*, 36: 129–144.

Milburn, T. (1994) 'Collaboration – It's the name of the game', *Concept*, 4: 13–15.

Millar, G. (1995) 'Beyond managerialism', *Youth and Policy*, 50: 49–58.

National Youth Agency (2004) *Ethical Conduct in Youth Work: A Statement of*

Values and Principles from the National Youth Agency, Leicester: The National Youth Agency.

Ranade, W. and Hudson, B. (2003) 'Conceptual issues in inter-agency collaboration', *Local Government Studies,* 29: 32–50.

Scottish Office (1996) *The Public Inquiry into the Shootings at Dunblane Primary School on 13th March 1996* (The Cullen Report), London: HMSO.

Smith, M. (1994) *Local Education*, Milton Keynes: Open University Press.

Tett, L. (2001) 'Collaborating for social justice: limits and possibilities for youth workers and schoolteachers in Scotland', *Education Links* (Australia), 61/62: 31–34.

Tett, L., Munn, P., Blair, A., Kay, H., Martin, I., Martin, J. and Ranson, S. (2001) 'Collaboration between schools and community education agencies in tackling social exclusion', *Research Papers in Education*, 16: 3–21.

Victor, B. and Cullen, J. (1988) 'The organisational bases of ethical work climates', *Administrative Science Quarterly,* 33: 101–125.

Weber, M. (1947) *The Theory of Social and Economic Organisation*, London: Oxford University Press.

Wenger, E. (1998) *Communities of Practice: Learning, Meaning and Identity*, Cambridge: Cambridge University Press.

Wilding, P. (1982) *Professional Power and Social Welfare*, London: Routledge & Kegan Paul.

Wilson, V. and Pirrie, A. (2001) *Multidisciplinary Team-working, Beyond the Barriers*, Edinburgh: SCRE.

4 Resourcing youth work

Dirty hands and tainted money

Tony Jeffs and Mark K. Smith

Introduction

Since youth work surfaced towards the end of the eighteenth century it has been strapped for cash. While uniformed and small local groups have frequently survived through voluntary effort, larger clubs, settlements and centres have habitually struggled to raise sufficient money and recruit enough volunteers to prosper. In this chapter we explore some key issues arising out of this need to secure funding. Our enquiry is based upon a review of the literature and interviews undertaken with managers and workers. We start by examining some of the tensions arising between philanthropic, state and commercial funding before looking at questions relating to funding sources, canvassing and fund-raising.

The volatility of youth work

An unremitting round of raising money, recruiting volunteers, gaining free or subsidised access to buildings and living with the prospect of imminent closure has been the norm for most youth organisations and groups. Even the few organisations and clubs that have survived for a century or more appear to encounter periods of crisis and retrenchment (see Jeffs and Gilchrist 2005). This seemingly inbuilt volatility is linked to a number of causes. First, there is the cyclical nature of membership with groups of young people affiliating and subsequently leaving when they believe they are 'too old' to belong or the attachment no longer meets a need. Second, changes take place in local neighbourhoods: for example, the changing profile of the population or a drift to the suburbs may result in clubs and organisations being 'stranded' in areas that are unable to provide a viable membership. Third, transformations in youth culture mean that once popular activities and forms of practice become *passé* and superfluous. Fourth, the centrality of personal relationships means that the loss of key workers or leaders can herald closure. Fifth, a weakening of the bonds of social solidarity in a locality can prefigure a possibly fatal decline in voluntary support and funding. Finally, economic and social changes impact upon youth work provision. For example, shifts in governmental funding priorities, growth in unemployment or a financial crisis can presage closure of youth projects. Social changes such as an upsurge in shift-working, a growth in commuting or a rise of home-based entertainment also impact heavily. Individually, and in permutation, these and other factors result in organisations failing or entering periods of crisis.

Problems are often approached as 'financial', but frequently finance is a symptom of other underlying issues. This said, loss of funding can and does precipitate the closure or weakening of popular, effective projects (Crimmens *et al.* 2004), since the best are as likely as the worst to be the victims of adjustments in the allocation of public sector funding or the financial failings of a voluntary organisation due to incompetent or dishonest management. Current funding structures in the public, private and voluntary sectors in no way operate to facilitate a Darwinian 'survival of the fittest', any more than our education system ensures that the most able climb to the top. Rather too often it is the lucky, even at times the most dishonest, who flourish at the expense of the best and most socially useful when funding is distributed according to political whim, bidding processes, commissioning or competitive tendering (Funnell *et al.* 2009; Newton 2006). Moreover, as we have moved from a youth work largely organised around the principle of young people contributing the bulk of the funding via membership fees, so they lose the influence which flows from that status (Jeffs 2001). Rather than being apprentice citizens exercising real control and influence they are demoted to the role of 'client', consumer or quasi-victim who is perhaps consulted about needs and services.

Philanthropy and the state

Historically much of the money (and labour) needed to sustain youth work has come from young people themselves, their parents and members of the immediate community (Jeffs and Smith 1988). In particular the role of faith organisations has been crucial in this respect, since it has long been the case that 'evangelicalism harnessed social conscience to liberal doctrine' (Prochaska 1988: 24; see also Prochaska 2006) and has operated in ways that favoured the development of youth work. With respect to philanthropic provision, one must acknowledge that this was never a top-down relationship, since from the beginning there was significant working-class involvement in religious and secular groups (Laqueur 1976; Smith 1988: 24–47).

Strong though the philanthropic impulse was, few youth workers questioned the desirability of state funding. Alternative sources were often capricious and fickle, as Robert Owen (founder of what was probably the first community education centre) and Hannah More (the Sunday School pioneer) discovered (Hopkins 1947: 185–195). Rich benefactors died, developed fresh interests or disliked youth workers' views and withdrew their backing. The same was true of the church leaders who controlled buildings. Hence More's advocacy of state funding: 'that the charity of the rich should ever be subsidiary to the public provision in those numberless instances to which the most equal laws cannot apply' (More, quoted in Collingwood and Collingwood 1990: 106). Others such as William Lovett (Lovett and Collins 1840), who promoted secular Chartist clubs and education programmes in the 1840s, saw democratically controlled state funding as a means of avoiding sectarian interference and of releasing education and self-help clubs from the clutches of those Thomas Carlyle dubbed the 'Aristocracy of the Moneybags'. A further argument for state involvement was developed by settlement and youth workers from the ideas of social idealists such as T.H. Green (Carter 2003; Plant 2006). Green viewed the state, in the right hands, as having the capacity to embrace superior moral characteristics to those which we might, in normal circumstances, encounter in the behaviour of the individual. The state could embody 'our higher self', a self more generous, caring and socially responsible than we might be in our daily lives. This philosophical position was indirectly transferred to a generation of public schoolboys and girls, with variable success, via an emphasis upon the importance of 'team spirit' and a need for Christians to communicate their faith through social service. This intellectual foundation provided an ideological bedrock upon which many boys' and girls' clubs, uniformed organisations and settlements were developed. Association, *esprit de corps* and sacrifice became ends and ideals. Predictably there were tensions, most notably around a fear that external funding might foster a dependency culture which would sabotage the efforts of workers to cultivate self-reliance. This was a view powerfully expressed by Octavia Hill, a pioneer of youth work and community action, who saw self-help and cooperation as the route to advancement for the working class (Hill 2005). Such trepidation was a minority position, as for most workers, state funding was viewed as a liberator. Welfare workers saw it as a means of making their jobs easier and allowing greater access to provision irrespective of a capacity to pay.

The rise of state funding

Once the principle of the state being the dominant provider of school and post-school education was accepted, state involvement in youth work became a foregone conclusion. From the late nineteenth century onward youth workers were among the shrill advocates of greater governmental interference in young people's lives (Hendrick 1990, 1994, 2001; Jeffs 1979). They were anxious that the same state that had deregulated the child and youth labour markets during the early years of industrialisation should once more do so and also fund universal schooling (Kirby 2003). Post-1918 there was negligible concern regarding the potential dangers of unrestrained state interference in youth work. A state monopoly of youth work first occurred in Communist Russia (Kelly 2007), then in Fascist Italy and finally by 1933 in Nazi Germany (Becker 1946; Knopp 2002) – a development which some youth organisations and educationalists welcomed (Feasey 1935; Stovin 1935). Post-1939 and the outbreak of war, advocacy of an all-embracing state youth service became muted. Instead a partnership of statutory and voluntary sectors emerged as the desired model, with a voluntary sector rooted in civil society being seen as a counterbalance to the centralising tendencies of state. Underpinning this concept was a covenant that central and local government would provide youth provision where the voluntary sector was unable to do so. Furthermore, governments recognised that for the partnership to succeed they must grant-aid some organisations and subsidise training. Aside from an ideological belief in the benefits of a mixed economy of welfare, self-interest sustained this compromise – since without voluntary provision, heightened demands for state investment in youth provision would arise.

Growth in state expenditure on youth work since 1945 has not followed a smoothly ascending trajectory. Between 1945 and 1959 it declined steeply, then rose sharply following publication of The Albemarle Report (HMSO 1960). Since then the changing economic fortunes and pressures on ministers to do 'something about the youth problem' have created peaks and troughs (Jeffs and Smith 1988, 1994, 2009; Stenson and Factor 1994, 1995; Cooper 2009). Since 1979 direct local authority expenditure on youth services has declined (Hawkins 1995; Maychell *et al.* 1996; Davies 2008) and been replaced by state funding mostly channelled through local authorities and other agencies. Normally these paymasters are 'commissioned' by central government to fund providers who are contracted to deliver specific pieces of work relating to, say, the arts, health promotion, environmental action, positive activities, school attendance or diversion from criminal activity.

Initially, like schools, 'statutory' youth work was financed by a mix of central government grants to local government and local taxation. The determination post-1979 of Conservative and New Labour governments in Britain to curtail local government and professional autonomy led to a dismantling of this arrangement. First, local authorities lost the capacity to set their own tax levels. Second, central government rechannelled resources from local education authorities (LEAs) to unelected quasi-governmental bodies such as development corporations and training and enterprise councils. These bodies then invited voluntary and statutory organisations, and subsequently private companies, to bid for these monies. Third, partially to compensate for cutbacks in LEA provision and to meet their own targets, statutory bodies such as police and health authorities began bankrolling non-formal education with young people. Finally, the government-licensed National Lottery has been used as an alternative means of funding youth work.

As a consequence of these changes, youth workers find themselves obligated to spend even more time raising money by bidding for project funding tied to given 'outcomes' and/or work with specified groups of young people. Whereas forty years ago a youth project with a full-time worker was predominately funded by a block grant or secondment from a local authority or charity (plus, in the case of clubs, income from membership fees), now it is usually reliant upon a plethora of grants, project money, ring-fenced funding and a sprinkling of charitable monies (see Gentleman 2009).

In addition, as commissioning and targets have taken hold, we have seen a growth in attempts to 'play the system'. As Seddon (2008: 10) has commented, public service workers have increasingly 'been "cheating" their systems to meet their targets'. The problem is that such 'cheating' or 'gaming' has become ubiquitous and endemic (Seddon 2008: 97). It arises directly out of systems organised around targets and delivery – and in the end can only be contained or eliminated by radically altering the basis upon which services are funded. A worrying effect of this is the extent to which these practices, which are, in effect, lying (Bok 1999), undermine the moral authority and integrity of frontline workers (Smith and Smith 2008: 142–144).

Thirty or forty years ago the ethical dilemmas relating to funding and expenditure might be encapsulated in the question 'How should I spend the money given by my employer (the local authority or charity) and the young people?' Now they are perhaps best summarised by the query 'What money should I or should I not bid for?' For each bid presents a fork in the road, an ethical dilemma that asks: 'Is it right for me to comply with the conditions that will be attached, or are they unacceptable?' This new funding structure has had a profound impact upon the agencies, as the manager of a homeless charity explains:

> The focus on getting the cash and delivering the contract takes attention away from the person who should matter the most to a charity: the beneficiary. The race for price cuts has tempted some charities to bid at levels they cannot in practice deliver, or to drive quality down below the point at which their service meets need.
>
> (Sampson 2009:1)

Ultimately, for many youth organisations and projects the quest for funding is resulting in a frantic privatised pursuit of self-interest wherein getting the money becomes more important than the doing. Consequently they are run in the interests of their own apparatchiks, not the young people or wider public. When this happens, survival and the balance sheet become the focus and end. Ethical considerations become irrelevant and the business model provides the paradigm and profit the compass.

Commercialisation and the 'new' youth work organisations

Coupled to these changes has been a series of initiatives aimed at creating a political and social climate that has reinforced the values of the free market and is hostile to collectivism. Governments have searched for ways of inserting free market values and competition into the management and delivery of services. A contract culture has been promoted whereby funding has had to be fought for. Finance is increasingly time-limited and dependent upon 'evidence' that a programme can deliver measurable outputs (Read 1996; Funnell *et al.* 2009). At a superficial level this ideological shift has led to the appearance of meaningless mission statements and charters pinned to club walls, members becoming customers and youth workers dressing up in the garb of the entrepreneur.

Complex philosophical factors are involved in changing from a youth worker to a chief executive; in moving to regarding oneself as an entrepreneur instead of a worker or a director rather than a team leader. Such mutations are more than mere semantics, or a by-product of changing fashions. They reflect conscious or unconscious choices as to how individuals or organisations perceive their role, and where they locate themselves on an ideological continuum. Growing commercialisation has, for example, 'forced' projects to secure business sponsorship as a precondition for receiving other monies, put advertising on the back of membership cards, and required representatives of the so-called business community to be appointed to management committees and governing bodies. These shifts have not occurred by accident. They flow, in part, from policy decisions made at the highest level. They are about ensuring that informal educators teach the values of the free market rather than collectivism, encourage greed not sacrifice, and consumption rather than restraint (Smith 2002). The contract culture operates a 'hidden hand' which imposes a harsh discipline. It brooks little opposition and because all are judged by vague and imprecise criteria it stifles criticism. One worker from a national voluntary agency reported that it 'has effectively silenced the voluntary sector. Line managers tell workers and they never argue about what they should prioritise.'

Alongside these changes we have witnessed in recent years the rise of new forms of youth work providers. These largely survive by securing local and central government contracts, most of which are time-limited and come with detailed targets and outcomes attached. Some are new providers established to exploit this market, others are long-established youth work organisations that have reorientated themselves to exploit the openings that exist through 'delivering' contracts. Whatever their background, all have strong business orientations and involve commercial interests more centrally in their management. Many attempt to encourage young people to see themselves as entrepreneurs and producers. Perhaps the most obvious examples of this arise in relation to projects around youth enterprise – but they also emerge in the arts and other fields. In addition, there are now a number of local agencies that specifically seek to develop the business acumen of young people and their ability to identify and exploit niche markets. Examples here include the provision of business units and support services; general education programmes around enterprise; money and support for business start-up and the formation of 'commercial arms' to produce and market goods and services such as furniture, videos, news items and environmental improvement.

A widespread feature is requiring young people to bid for funding and enter into competition with other groups of young people to secure resources or access to help. Another characteristic tends to be an emphasis on developing, promoting and selling a 'distinctive' product or service often linked to a given issue such as sexual health or 'positive activities' to schools or local authorities. Some individual workers have also entered this arena – developing services that can be bought in by youth work providers. It then becomes a small step into the provision of play and youth work services that are for profit. Examples of this are common within the field of 'leisure-time animation' in Italy and France (Lorenz 1994: 101), but there are also substantial initiatives in the UK, for example, in the commercial provision of adventure holidays, and of play opportunities in shopping malls. This is likely to be an area of some growth, with fast food chains such as MacDonald's, leisure providers such as Warner Brothers and 'lifestyle' companies seeking new markets close to their core businesses. What sets this form of 'youth work' apart is that it is 'market led' and not responsive to the expressed or observed needs of the young people. Furthermore, given that the funding is outcome led, although artificial attempts to build in consultation and participation may be included in the contract specifications, the focus and direction of the work is predetermined.

These changes regarding how youth work is oriented and funded require workers to confront some difficult ethical dilemmas in relation to three interlinked questions:

- Should agencies actively canvass for funding?
- Are certain sources of funding ethically unacceptable?
- Are certain methods of collecting/obtaining funding ethically unacceptable?

We now consider each of these – examining how workers have tried to make sense of practice in relation to ideas about what makes for 'the good' for human beings.

Should agencies and workers actively canvas for funding?

Should youth organisations seek external money? Some workers have argued that to do so exposes them to accusations of self-interest and an absence of faith. Typical of these were Georg Müller in England and William Quarrier in Scotland (who were both involved in developing orphanages and young people's communities). Each saw their work as revealing the will of God. They postulated that as long as they followed His direction all would be well:

> The work was the Lord's and William Quarrier only his agent. God would provide. Accordingly there never was an appeal for money, no bazaars to raise funds, no envelope collection. It was an enterprise in faith from the beginning.
>
> (Ross 1971: 13)

Müller likewise never pleaded for or solicited funds (Pierson 1902). Thomas Barnardo had scant patience for such individuals, describing them as a 'race of philanthropists and Evangelists who live on faith and postage stamps' (quoted in Wagner 1979: 198). Today when the chase for funding often seems all-consuming, it is worth reflecting on this position. Some still hold to the principle of not soliciting funding, as one explained: 'if the work is worth doing then the resources will be found'. He described how individuals and church organisations sustained his work with young people with unsolicited gifts and donations. He made it a principle never to ask or bid for funding, arguing that the important thing is do the right thing according to your values and to see the young people as active agents rather than as passive consumers who if given the opportunity would do far more for themselves.

Many workers are being forced to devote ever more time to fund-raising at the expense of face-to-face work. Of course some prefer attending fund-raising events, writing letters and mixing with 'movers and shakers' to the company of young people and the local community. Others recognise what is happening and resent it, yet a sense of duty drives them on. Eventually a question is likely to arise for many youth projects that are 'contract dependent' regarding whether they are undertaking this or that piece of work because it has intrinsic value for young people or because it keeps worker X or Y in a job or a building open. At what point does the work become self-serving rather than socially useful?

The question here is less whether active canvassing is wrong and more about the extent. How do workers make judgements regarding this? Do they confine themselves to seeking out core or essential funding or do they simply view fund-raising as a fact of life? One 'solution' favoured by Breen (1993: 158) was to look to young people. He abandoned the centre which consumed all his time and energy to maintain and left him too exhausted to 'concentrate on relationships'. Rather than worry about buildings and resources, he insisted that if the young people you work with want money for a project or somewhere to meet, they will, and indeed must, perhaps with your help, secure these resources for themselves. For Breen the role of the worker is not dispenser of resources which inevitably creates a 'provider–client' relationship and 'patronising attitudes' (Breen 1993: 50) but to be an educator, friend and ally. This approach still leaves important ethical questions. Who should they accept money from, what strings should be attached, and how much effort should they put into the activity?

Robert Woods, the pioneer American settlement and club worker, viewed dependency on philanthropy as an ever-present threat, encouraging workers to avoid the difficult task of engaging with the community and involving local people. Instead it motivated them to devote their attention to the wealthy who could endow the club with money and overlook the poor who could only offer their time and talents. Therefore, to:

> canvass for money would be as much against our principles as a canvass for information, and I think it would be better to get acquainted gradually with local citizens and to educate them by object lessons as to their duty.
>
> (Woods 1929: 68)

Few would risk adopting the approach of Quarrier, Breen and Woods. The interviewee who informed us he never bothered seeking '£500 from Mr and Mrs Bloggs, I am looking for big money and want to get in with the big players' would surely have little sympathy with it. Yet many reading this could compile a list of projects where dangerous confusion has arisen regarding ends and means. The result can be that staff invest disproportionate energy and resources in sustaining the project, the building or their own salaries at the expense of the needs of the clientele. They may well exploit young people and other workers in doing so. Refusing to solicit for funding is one way to avoid this temptation and dilemma. It will not of course eliminate such temptation but it can encourage a much clearer focus on the role and purpose of the work.

Are certain sources of funding ethically unacceptable?

Many workers have grappled with questions such as 'How can we fund our work without subverting the values which underpinned it?' A nun working with homeless young people recounted such a tension. She saw the work as 'helping people to value themselves, to feel at peace with who they are, to recognise their worth and gifts and creating opportunities for them to contribute'. She continued:

> I resist talking of the work as a 'project' and I try to avoid chasing money as I feel it is so easy to get caught in that trap and in the latest trends. I get people telling me about the sources of money and they seemed surprised when I seem not to be interested . . . I just wonder if we could just become like everyone else in the sense of moving into 'in' areas of work, where the money is. This shouldn't be what we are about. I think we must be distinctive in the sense we are part of the wider church, of the transcendent, part of working for something bigger, standing for a set of values and principles, centred on the Gospel and not on the market or state.

She also described the disbelief bordering on outrage when she suggested to colleagues and supporters that they should no longer be a registered charity. She argued that such a status demeaned and stigmatised those with whom they worked and created in the minds of the workers a false perception of their role.

Even where organisations have refused to canvas or chase funding, they are still left with the question of what money to accept and what to refuse. In our review three key questions emerged:

- Does taking money from certain sources seriously undermine the moral authority of the workers?
- Does the form which funding takes stigmatise young people?
- Are the 'strings' attached acceptable?

Sources of funding and the moral authority of workers

In 1891 after working at Hull House (a settlement in Chicago) for a number of years with a group of young women, Jane Addams perceived the need for a girls' club linked to the settlement but with its own building. After sharing this with colleagues and supporters, a trustee informed Addams that a friend had offered the $20,000 required to open a clubhouse. Subsequently she learned that the prospective donor was a man notorious for underpaying the young women in his establishment and about whom 'even darker stories' were circulating. Following heated exchanges among trustees, staff and members, the donation was dubbed 'tainted money' and returned. Her position was that:

> social changes can only be inaugurated by those who feel the unrighteousness of contemporary conditions, and the expression of their scruples may be one opportunity for pushing forward moral tests into that dubious area wherein wealth is accumulated.
>
> (Addams 1930: 139)

Addams was not alone in adopting this stance. Lilian Wald, founder of the Henry Street Settlement in New York, who was a pacifist, objected in 1916 to the trustees investing in Bethlehem Steel, a company that was profiting from war orders.

According to Carson the majority of American settlement and club workers during this period did not share the position of Wald and Addams. Not only did they refrain from questioning the origins of a donation but they also tempered campaigns against sweated labour, slum landlords and political corruption to avoid offending 'prosperous and often "conservative" uptown patrons' (Carson 1990: 53). The latter group came to dominate, and the issue of 'tainted money', which attracted so much attention within the settlement and club movement in America around the turn of the century, faded from view.

Certain religious groups have, however, consistently avoided taking money from specific sources. As a worker related, 'because it is a Methodist church . . . you couldn't apply to somewhere like a brewery, or somewhere to do with tobacco. Also you can't apply to certain lotteries.' It is not only agencies controlled by certain religious bodies which have to negotiate this issue. We were told of an ecumenical youth housing project that withdrew a National Lottery bid, despite a serious risk that it would fold, because the long-standing representative of the Baptist Church on the steering group said she would resign if they proceeded. The money was raised from elsewhere, as the majority of the steering group held that her departure would compromise the project's ecumenical ethos. Others construct somewhat tenuous ways of getting around their principles. One Methodist centre, for example, agreed in relation to National Lottery monies: 'you can't apply for money to do things to the building . . . but you can for a project that directly tackles poverty'.

Some are unequivocal regarding their position. A representative of the Girls' Brigade explained why they would not accept Lottery funds:

> We exist to offer girls a Christian viewpoint on life and it would be completely inconsistent to teach them to value and serve other people while the organisation itself accepted funding from a source where people can only gain by the loss of others.
>
> (quoted in Tondeur 1996: 132)

The debate regarding whether or not National Lottery funding is acceptable has predominately been shaped by competing religious positions around gambling (Tondeur 1996; see also Perkins 1933). Yet the discussion has implications for all workers, and serves as a contemporary example of the 'tainted money' predicament, since it requires workers to consider how acceptance might undermine their moral authority. Does receipt of Lottery funding help to legitimise participation in this and other forms of gambling? It is impossible to envisage a youth club trip to a casino being sanctioned by management, or a worker teaching young people how to fill in a betting slip being allowed to keep their post. Evidence indicates that between 5 and 7 per cent of young people are 'problem gamblers' (Griffith 2003; Valentine 2008) and that the National Lottery and scratch cards play a substantive role in encouraging gambling among young people (Griffith 2003; Wood and Griffiths 2002). For youth workers and teachers to point a disapproving finger at such shopkeepers smacks of hypocrisy. Their eagerness to grab a share of the profits from such sales, and the unashamed way in which many boast of their 'success' in securing Lottery spoils, make it impossible for them to continue to express disapproval of gambling among the young. Consequently organisers of the UK National Lottery have sought respectability by aligning with good causes to put 'clear blue water' between itself and what it hopes will become classified as less reputable forms of gambling. Predictably it targets youth organisations to both tempt future customers and because 'young people' and youthful activities bestow a clean, healthy image.

National Lottery funding is not of itself 'tainted money'. Those who enjoy a flutter at the racecourse or see a poker-school as a place where skills are exercised and social networks forged may with justification sneer at the intellectual vacuum at the heart of the proceedings but can scarcely judge the resulting handouts as tainted. However, those who seek to discourage gambling in the young will find it difficult to do otherwise. Sadly, the growing dependency of youth organisations upon National Lottery funds has not stimulated a serious discussion concerning either the place of gambling within youth work or the case for or against retaining prohibitions which prevent young people from gambling.

At specific times some groups have sought to disassociate themselves from potential sponsors. For a period Barclays Bank was boycotted by student unions and a number of community projects because of its links with the apartheid regime in South Africa. Nestlé was similarly treated owing to its policy of marketing baby milk products in developing countries. However, in the sometimes murky world of charity fund-raising the spectre of a company with such public relations difficulties has acted as a spur to an approach by an agency. Companies such as BP and Shell, which from time to time hit problems with environmental groups, have been quick to put money into environmental projects aimed at young people and to advertise this fact. Without exception, those interviewed said they would decline a donation from a cigarette company. Cynics might point out that, unlike the National Lottery, cigarette manufacturers, major environmental polluters and exploiters of third world child labour, such as the leading manufacturers of sporting goods, have never sponsored youth work on any scale, so disapproval requires no sacrifice.

Does stigmatisation result?

In raising money there is a tendency to paint an exaggerated image of young people both as victims, needing help, and a threat to society, needing to be managed. Several workers voiced their concern about the way in which young people apparently have to be presented to gain funding. Over the years there has been a fairly consistent appeal to moral panics as a way of selling youth work (Jeffs and Smith 1988: 14–40). As a local authority youth work adviser commented: 'If you want money it is now a matter of promising to do something about crime or graffiti to get your hands on it.'

Whether it is youth crime, sexual health, drug addiction or school under-achievement, fears about these issues can be appealed to and youth work offered as part of a solution. The result has been a series of funding initiatives that target particular behaviours and groups. To access such money, agencies must 'fit' those with whom they work, or seek to work with, into sets of often stereotypical and sometimes demeaning categories. If they gain funding, workers justify what they have done in relation to the same problematic categories. The result can be either a subversion of the work – typically at the moment involving a pandering to authoritarianism (Jeffs and Smith 1994; Cooper 2009) – or problems in reporting. The latter can entail straightforward lying or presenting work in alternative ways (which may not be to the satisfaction of the funder). As one worker put it:

> I realise that some colouring of the facts might be necessary to get money for this community, but it is getting ridiculous. To get . . . [some funding] . . . I now have a choice: change the way I work or lie.

A further fear is that by participating in such categorisation, youth work organisations confirm a picture of young people as thugs, victims or users. Their work is presented to funders as helping to 'solve' a problem relating to young people. Simultaneously, this strengthens a popular prejudice and undermines practices that may have strengthened those young people's sense of worth and possibility.

Conditions and strings

Issues concerning the strings attached to funding can relate to the way in which young people are presented to the sorts of activities that may be involved, and to practical issues around when and how money may be spent. However, there have been persistent worries around conditions concerning the direction which youth work takes. Considerable discussion has occurred regarding the extent to which a worker can legitimately seek to change the lifestyle or beliefs of young people. Controversy has centred on matters of faith and patriotism. Some organisations have been open regarding their determination to convert. As a founder of the YWCA explained, a central role was to release girls 'enchained by Judaism, Popery, and heathenism' (quoted in Moor 1910: 244). Yet flagrant attempts to train and convert are difficult to square with the role of the youth worker as educator. As Peters (1966: 203) argues, the function of the educator is to initiate young people 'into skill, attitudes and knowledge which are necessary for them to participate intelligently as citizens of a democratic state' and not to act 'as a missionary for any church or as a recruiting officer for any political party'.

Loss of empire and the professionalisation of the armed forces has virtually eradicated pressure on youth workers to prepare young people for military service, while the declining influence of religious bodies in public life has generally liberated those not directly employed by them from the role of missionary. Indeed the pendulum has swung in the opposite direction: those who seek to convert young people risk dismissal from most secular agencies.

Nowadays, pressure to serve as a missionary or recruiting sergeant has been supplanted by coercion to perform as a huckster for particular brands and products. Multinational companies and local rivals increasingly target educational agencies not to ensure that they produce the 'perfect' worker but compliant 'dumbed-down' consumers (Barber 2007). Youth workers are, like other educators, being bribed to create marketing opportunities for firms anxious to capture consumers while they are of an 'impressionable age'. They are being 'persuaded', in return for sponsorship, to endorse products by putting up adverts in centres; adding company logos to membership cards, reports, leaflets and notepaper; and promoting marketing ploys such as discount cards. It is a system which not only enables corporations to target advertising but equally the payment secures them the tacit endorsement of a youth organisation with a reputation for probity and generates '700,000 trustworthy, walking advertisements' (Tran 1990: 6; see also Giroux 2000).

In the nineteenth century a compliant government encouraged religious organisations to corrupt the educational process by restricting the access of young people to open dialogue, honest debate and untainted knowledge. Today, equally supine politicians encourage business organisations to do the same. Whereas their predecessors usually had the excuse that they sincerely believed they were saving the souls of the young, now greed provides the motive for the donors, and a craven desire to cut public spending serves as the political justification. To this has been added a further issue. Some agencies are selling the young people with whom they work as marketing opportunities. In the United States, in return for cash, thousands of schools have installed televisions tuned to a predetermined station in classrooms, corridors and canteens. These pump out adverts and promotional material aimed at young people who cannot choose an alternative programme or switch it off and, because attendance is compulsory, have no choice but to watch it (Apple 1993; Kenway and Bullen 2001). In the UK firms such as Tesco have effectively used schools and other educational agencies to bring moral pressure on children and their parents to shop in their stores – greatly to the profit of the store – by issuing tokens exchangeable for equipment (Hoggart 1995: 32).

Sponsorship also leads to young people and youth workers being used as billboards. Payment often requires them to wear T-shirts and hats advertising particular products or the names of their sponsors. Arguing that we should not worry unduly because young people are too sophisticated to be taken in ignores the research of the advertisers which tells them who to target and independent investigations which confirm not only that young people are susceptible to advertising but that it is the least well educated who are the most vulnerable (Balding *et al.* 1996). For youth workers, and indeed all educators, advertising is something that must be recognised as an adversary of truth, 'a form of discourse where only the best side of a case is put forward' (Young 1990: 291) and the vices are deliberately hidden. Advertising is a teller of 'fictional tales' (Williams 1980), and as such, serious ethical concern must emanate from any attempt to allow it to wheedle its way into the youth work environment. One may be unable to exclude it, any more than one can keep out sexism or violence, but that does not justify inviting it in.

Are certain methods of gaining funding ethically unacceptable?

Many youth organisations pay considerable attention to the 'how' of raising income. At the centre of this concern may be a desire to ensure that the methods employed avoid subverting the moral values and teachings of the organisation. There is also the hope that young people will learn socially useful lessons from involvement in the process of collection. As might be expected, the importance of consistency is stressed since, as Barrow (1975: 52) points out, if an educator or leader says you should do this then they are committing themselves to the view that they and those whom they teach 'ought also to do this in the same circumstances'. As Colquhoun (1954: 68) explained, the Scout Law set the highest possible standard for boys to aspire to. Therefore, all those connected to the organisation must set themselves a 'higher standard in regard to methods of raising money than others do' (Colquhoun 1954: 68). Indeed, the rules of the Scout Movement state: 'money should be earned and not solicited' (ibid.: 69). Henriques (1933: 111) was similarly determined that within the Boys' Club Movement all those involved should contribute something, since:

> anything that savours of charity in the minds of the boys is obnoxious and distasteful to the highest degree . . . all boys must contribute, 'pauperization in a boys' club is loathsome'.

Avoidance of begging reflects a desire not to exploit the young people. Traditionally this has been interpreted as not using their labour to sustain an organisation which has been established to serve them. This, for example, was the basis of the objections voiced within the Boys' Brigade to the launching in 1921 of B-B Week when members were sent out to raise money. Although these criticisms were set aside, it still remains to this day an area of contention within some organisations. It is generally assumed that although young people should make some financial contribution in order to give them a stake and avoid 'pauperization', this should be more than balanced by a contribution from elsewhere.

The examples of sponsorship discussed not only exploit young people but corrupt the educational process. As a worker pointed out, all too often it means that 'projects have to be constructed around what will attract sponsorship rather than what we as workers choose to believe is needed'. This also leads to the expressed needs of the young people being relegated to the margins. Another said: 'Unless we find an alternative . . . then our young people will be locked into a slavery of intellect and a servility of attitude.'

A further set of questions arises around the way in which many youth organisations have enthusiastically embraced business interests and partners. In the New Youth Work Organisations there tends to be less of a tension between their expressed aims and their mode of operation. If they see themselves as businesses then it is fairly easy and consistent to view young people as customers. Within those local authorities and agencies that have gone down the 'charter' and 'commissioning' route there has been significant pressure from the centre to promote 'customer care' and 'customer satisfaction'. The problem for youth work is that this involves a fundamental misreading of both the educational process and the ultimate aims of the work. To view young people as consumers is to see them essentially as objects to be acted upon. Like pizzas, services are 'delivered' to them. If we are to approach the work in a proper educational spirit, then, rather than being consumers, young people need to be engaged with as active participants, creators of their own meanings and possibilities.

Conclusion

An inevitable consequence of the voluntary nature of the relationship between young people and youth workers is that the latter, perhaps more than most educators, rely on their moral authority to secure a constituency. Securing and retaining such authority, often in trying circumstances, creates an ever-present tension within the work since, without resorting to subterfuge, they must seek to become the kind of people young people 'can trust, both intellectually and with regard to their character . . . steady, completely reliable and consistent' (Warnock 1993: 23). Consequently they must pay careful attention to their reputation. How an organisation raises its income tells us a great deal about underpinning values and ethics. As the young people affiliated to an organisation are likely to be aware of where the money comes from and how it was raised (indeed, they often help to procure it), workers can never totally side-step the questions raised here regarding whether agencies should actively canvas for funding and whether certain sources of funding and particular methods of collecting/obtaining it are ethically unacceptable.

Current funding arrangements disadvantage those who seek to operate according to ethical considerations. Part of the problem is that many funders have not considered these sorts of ethical questions. As one agency manager explained:

> these people hadn't thought about the issues until we went and asked them about funding. The ethical dimension had simply been absent.

However, many agencies are also guilty of the same omission. As one of the interviewees commented, many 'hadn't thought about the issues around funding until we went and asked'.

Just how workers and agencies can be encouraged to consider ethical questions is open to debate. Some may want to go down the route of writing a policy statement (in much the same way that equal opportunities statements have appeared). However, adoption of policy statements can mean little unless the questions approached are wrestled with and those who create them have sincere intentions to live by the values embodied in them. Enron, a company that systematically cheated its employees, investors and customers, had a code of ethics over sixty pages long that 'was a model of its kind' (Newton 2006: 16). Many youth work agencies, although they do not set out to behave immorally or fraudulently, also produce mission statements and codes of ethics that have as little impact on the daily practice as Enron's did. Far more important than concocting vague statements is the need to examine practice through an ethical lens, and to pay much-needed attention to exploring what might make for the good in practice. The current technical focus on measurable outcomes and competencies tends towards the 'correct' rather than what is 'right' (see Jeffs and Smith 2008, and 1990: 17–18, 124–143). This disposition to 'rule-following' and safety first tends to sideline active consideration of what might be good – and as such is anti-educational. Engaging with ethical questions around funding, and involving people within that conversation, is a central task for workers and agencies. Without it, claims to moral authority wither away.

Questions for reflection and discussion

1   What, if any, suppliers of goods or services would you deem to be ethically unacceptable as sponsors of youth work projects? How would you justify this?

2   Imagine you are a youth worker in a situation where a company sponsoring a residential weekend expected participants to wear a T-shirt or hat sporting their logo. Would you enforce that expectation? What would you say to a young person who refused? Would you be willing to accept money on condition that you wore items bearing a sponsor's logo during your working hours?

Recommended reading

Barber, B.R. (2007) Con$umed: How Markets Corrupt Children, Infantilize Adults, and Swallow Citizens Whole, New York: W.W. Norton. This book shows how adults are infantilised in a global economy that overproduces goods and targets children as consumers.

Giroux, H.A. (2000) *Stealing Innocence: Youth, Corporate Power, and the Politics of Culture*, New York: St Martin's Press. This book explores the way in which corporate culture is encroaching on children's and young people's lives.

Jeffs, T. and Smith, M.K. (2008) 'Valuing youth work', *Youth and Policy*, 100: 277–302. This article gives an overview of the nature and value of youth work in a changing climate of policy and practice.

Acknowledgements

We wish to express our gratitude to those who allowed themselves to be interviewed and to those who helped us do the interviewing: Phil Watson, Sarah Hackett, Nathan Ward and Huw Blacker.

References

Addams, J. (1930) *Twenty Years at Hull House*, New York: Macmillan.

Apple, M. (1993) *Official Knowledge: Democratic Education in a Conservative Age*, New York: Routledge.

Balding, J., Regis, D., Wise, A., Bish, D. and Muirden, J. (1996) *Bully Off: Young People that Fear Going to School*, Exeter: Schools Health Education Unit, University of Exeter.

Barber, B.R. (2007) *Con$umed: How Markets Corrupt Children, Infantilize Adults, and Swallow Citizens Whole*, New York: W.W. Norton.

Barrow, R. (1975) *Moral Philosophy for Education*, London: Unwin.

Becker, H. (1946) *German Youth: Bond or Free?*, London: RKP.

Bok, S. (1999) *Lying: Moral Choice and Public and Private Life*, New York: Vintage.

Breen, M. (1993) *Outside In: Reaching Unreached Young People Today*, London: Scripture Union.

Carson, M. (1990) *Settlement Folk: Social Thought and the American Settlement Movement 1885–1930*, Chicago, IL: University of Chicago Press.

Carter, M. (2003) *T.H. Green and the Development of Ethical Socialism*, Thorverton: Academic Imprint.

Collingwood, J. and Collingwood, M. (1990) *Hannah More*, Oxford: Lion Publishers.

Colquhoun, J.F. (1954) *Running a Scout Troop*, London: Boy Scout Association.

Cooper, C. (2009) 'Rethinking the "problem of youth"', *Youth and Policy*, 104: 48–60.

Crimmens, D., Factor, F., Jeffs, T., Pitts, J., Pugh, C., Spence, J. and Turner, P. (2004) *Reaching Socially Excluded Young People: A National Study of Street-based Youth Work*, York: Joseph Rowntree Foundation.

Davies, B. (2008) *The New Labour Years: A History of the Youth Service Volume 3 1997–2007*, Leicester: National Youth Agency.

Feasey, L. (1935) 'Authority and individuality in European education today', *The New Era in Home and School*, October.

Funnell, W., Jupe, R. and Andrew, J. (2009) *In Government We Trust: Market Failure and the Decisions of Privatisation*, Sydney: UNSW Press.

Gentleman, A. (2009) 'Lost in nowhere land', *Guardian*, 15 July: 3.

Giroux, H.A. (2000) *Stealing Innocence: Youth, Corporate Power, and the Politics of Culture*, New York: St Martin's Press.

Griffith, D. (2003) 'Adolescent Gambling: risk factors and simplifications for prevention, intervention and treatment' in D. Romer (ed.) *Reducing Adolescent Risk: towards an integrated approach*, Thousand Oaks, CA: Sage.

Griffiths, M. (2002) *Gambling and Gambling Addictions in Adolescence*, Leicester: British Psychological Society/Blackwell.

Hawkins, P. (1995) *Formula Funding and Financial Delegation in Youth Services and Adult Education*, Leicester: Youth Work Press.

Hendrick, H. (1990) *Images of Youth: Age, Class and the Male Youth Problem 1880–1920*, Oxford: Clarendon Press.

Hendrick, H. (1994) *Child Welfare in England 1872–1989*, London: Routledge.

Hendrick, H. (2001) *Children Childhood and English Society 1880–1990*, Bristol: Policy Press.

Henriques, B. (1933) *Club Leadership*, London: Oxford University Press.

HMSO (1960) *The Youth Service in England and Wales* (The Albemarle Report), London: HMSO.

Hill, O. (2005) *Octavia Hill's Letters to Fellow Workers, 1872–1911: Together with an Account of the Walmer Street Industrial Experiment* (edited by R. Whelan), London: Kyrle Books.

Hoggart, R. (1995) *The Way We Live Now*, London: Chatto & Windus.

Hopkins, M.A. (1947) *Hannah More and her Circle*, New York: Longmans, Green & Co.

Jeffs, A.J. (1979) *Young People and the Youth Service*, London: RKP.

Jeffs, T. (2001) 'Citizenship, youth work and democratic renewal', *Scottish Youth Issues Journal*, 3: 11–34.

Jeffs, T. and Gilchrist, R. (2005) *Newcastle YMCA: 150 Years*, Newcastle: Newcastle YMCA/The National Youth Agency.

Jeffs, T. and Smith, M. (1988) 'The political economy of youth work', in T. Jeffs and M. Smith (eds) *Welfare and Youth Work Practice*, London: Macmillan.

—— (eds) (1990) *Using Informal Education: An Alternative to Casework, Teaching and Control?*, Buckingham: Open University Press.

—— (1994) 'Young people, youth work and a new authoritarianism', *Youth and Policy*, 46: 17–32.

—— (2008) 'Valuing youth work', *Youth and Policy*, 100: 277–302.

—— (eds) (2009) *Youth Work: Policy and Practice*, Basingstoke: Palgrave.

Kelly, C. (2007) *Children's World: Growing Up in Russia 1890–1991*, New Haven, CN: Yale University Press.

Kenway, J. and Bullen, E. (2001) *Consuming Children: Education-entertainment-advertising*, Buckingham: Open University Press.

Knopp, G. (2002) *Hitler's Children*, Stroud: Sutton Publishing.

Kirby, P. (2003) *Child Labour in Britain, 1750–1870*, Basingstoke: Palgrave Macmillan.

Laqueur, T.W. (1976) *Religion and Respectability: Sunday Schools and Working Class Culture*, New Haven, CT: Yale University Press.

Lorenz, W. (1994) *Social Work in a Changing Europe*, London: Routledge.

Lovett, W. and Collins, J. (1840) *Chartism: A new organization of the people: embracing a plan for the education and improvement of the people, politically and socially . . . written in Warwick gaol*, London: J. Watson.

Maychell, K., Pathak, S. and Cato, V. (1996) *Providing for Young People: Local Authority Youth Services in the 1990s*, Slough: NFER.

Moor, L.M. (1910) *Girls of Yesterday and Today: The Romance of the YWCA*, London: S.W. Partridge.

Newton, L.H. (2006) *Permission to Steal: Revealing the Roots of Corporate Scandal*, Oxford: Blackwell.

Perkins, E. Benson (1933) *Gambling and Youth*, London: National Sunday School Union.

Peters, R.S. (1966) *Ethics and Education*, London: Unwin.

Pierson, A.T. (1902) *George Müller of Bristol*, London: Pickering and Inglis.

Plant, R. (2006) 'T.H. Green: citizenship, education and the law', *Oxford Review of Education*, 32: 23–37.

Prochaska, F. (1988) *The Voluntary Impulse. Philanthropy in Modern Britain*, London: Faber and Faber.

Prochaska, F. (2006). *Christianity and Social Service in Modern Britain: The Disinherited Spirit*, Oxford: Oxford University Press.

Read, P. (1996) 'A quest for funding' , *Young People Now*, 89: 24–25.

Ross, J. (1971) *The Power I Pledge: A Study of the Life of William Quarrier*, Bridge of Weir: Quarrier's Homes.

Seddon, J. (2008) *Systems Thinking in the Public Sector: The Failure of the Reform Regime – and the Manifesto for a Better Way*, Axminster: Triarchy.

Smith, M. (1988) *Developing Youth Work: Informal Education, Mutual Aid and Popular Practice*, Milton Keynes: Open University Press.

Smith, M.K. (2002) 'Globalization and the incorporation of education', *The Encyclopedia of Informal Education*, www.infed.org/biblio/globalization.htm (accessed 15 September 2009).

Smith, H. and Smith, M.K. (2008) *The Art of Helping Others: Being Around, Being There, Being Wise*, London: Jessica Kingsley.

Stenson, K. and Factor, F. (1994) 'Youth work, risk and crime prevention', *Youth and Policy*, 46: 1–15.

Stenson, K. and Factor, F. (1995) 'Governing youth: new directions for the youth service', in J. Baldock and M. May (eds) *Social Policy Review 7*, Canterbury: Social Policy Association.

Stovin, H. (1935) *Totem: The Exploitation of Youth*, London: Methuen.

Tondeur, K. (1996) *What Price the Lottery?*, Crowborough: Monarch Publications.

Tran, M. (1990) 'Keep Boy Scouts pure', *Guardian*, 31 December: 6.

Valentine, G. (2008) *Literature Review of Children and Young People's Gambling*, London: Gambling Commission.

Wagner, G. (1979) *Barnardo*, London: Weidenfeld & Nicolson.

Warnock, M. (1993) 'Good teaching', in R. Barrow and P. White (eds) *Beyond Liberal Education: Essays in Honour of Paul H. Hirst,* London: Routledge.

Williams, R. (1980) *Problems in Materialism and Culture: Selected Essays,* London: Verso.

Wood, R. and Griffiths, M. (2002) 'Adolescent perceptions of the National Lottery and scratch cards: a qualitative study using group interviews', *Journal of Adolescence,* 25: 655–668.

Woods, E.H. (1929) *Robert A Woods: A Biography,* Cambridge, MA: Riverside Press.

Young, B.M. (1990) *Television Advertising and Children,* Oxford: Clarendon Press.

Part 2
Ethical issues in practice

5 Youth workers as professionals

Managing dual relationships and maintaining boundaries

Howard Sercombe

Introduction

The 'dual relationships problem' is a term used across the professions to talk about potential difficulties that can arise when a practitioner has a professional relationship with someone, but also another kind of relationship with the same person which has different (and perhaps conflicting) obligations and expectations (Corey *et al.* 2007). The problem was first identified in the ethics of medicine, around treating a family member: the concern was that strong emotional feelings might impair professional judgement and decision-making (Cook and Hoas 2001). However, it is just as important in youth work. A young person may work at the hair salon which a youth worker uses, or go to their church, or routinely end up at the same nightclub. In these situations, the roles and rules can easily become confused (Gottlieb 1993), and the boundaries start to shift and become uncertain. The sites where this may emerge are expanding all the time with the advent of social networking sites and the possibility of out-of-work 'friend'-type contacts online.

This chapter will outline some typical situations involving dual relationships, explore what can go wrong in such situations, and offer guidance on how to minimise problems when dual relationships cannot be avoided.

Background

There are certain characteristics of youth work as a profession which sometimes make the boundaries difficult to specify and difficult for young people to recognise. The informal nature of youth work means that often there is no space or time boundary around the action: it is not a fifty-minute consultation in a counselling room with the door closed. The youth work relationship can feel like a friendship, with lots of the elements of friendship such as good-natured ribbing and play. Language codes are often those that the young people use, so it can feel to them and to the youth worker as if that worker is one of the gang.

In such a context, youth workers need to be clear about the nature of their relationship, and especially the limits of that relationship. Lack of clarity can easily lead to conflicts of interest, real ethical dilemmas and a sense of betrayal from young people when expectations are disappointed. This relates both to *roles*: what kind of relationship template (for example, friend, mother, confidante, teacher, peer group leader) is projected and reproduced in the relationship, and *domains*: what will be the limits in different aspects of the relationship (such as time, space, money, emotional connection, availability). These interconnect, so that certain role templates will project certain domain boundaries and expectations. Friends, for example, are generally available to each other in leisure time. In professional relationships, people are not generally available to each other in leisure time. Family creates obligations regardless of affinity (that is, whether or not family members like each other): friendship does not.

There are a number of settings in which dual relationships can arise. It is not unusual in Britain for youth workers to start off as members of youth clubs, become volunteers, and then members of staff. In this case, youth workers may be working with members of what used to be their own peer group. In some circumstances, young people could be members of a youth worker's extended family: cousins, nieces, nephews, younger brothers and sisters, the sons and daughters of friends, or perhaps worse, of employers. A person who was a participant in a youth activity yesterday may be a team mate on a sporting team today and a drinking companion down at the local pub after the game tonight – or their parents might. This is common when youth workers are part of the community in which they are working, such as small country towns, and therefore have multiple loyalties and obligations. Multiple relationships cannot be avoided there, because there are more roles than people, and everyone is taking part in a range of activities. There is often limited choice. In the city, youth workers can choose to go to a different pub than the one frequented by the young people they work with, or shop at a different store from the one a young person works at. Youth workers can get their plumbing fixed by someone other than a young person's father. In small communities, there may not be that choice (Schank and Skovholt 1997; Sercombe 2006; Younggren 2003).

Communities of difference, such as the LGBT (lesbian, gay, bisexual or transgender) community, or ethnic or cultural communities, may have some similar characteristics. Everyone knows each other and is involved in multiple roles in the relationships they have. A youth worker's priest or imam may be their uncle too: and he might be the only priest/imam in the community. Some communities, such as Aboriginal communities, are *defined* by kin relationships: a person's identity only makes sense as a member of the community if they have a family connection, and if they do not, one will be invented for them. It is the relationship that makes them part of the community.

Youth accommodation settings, unless well thought out and well designed, can be thick with dual relationship situations, especially where a young person is living with a worker in their home. In general, this is frowned upon in youth work circles, but there is no clear consensus about it, especially in faith-based work. The worker is then a parent figure, a housemate, or a landlord or landlady, as well as their youth worker.

Role approximation

A history of contact with youth workers may not be every young person's experience. They may never have met a youth worker before, so will have to work to make sense of the relationship. If the youth worker is not crystal clear about the nature of youth work practice, and is messy in their conception of the relationship, you can expect the young person to be the same.

The standard way people work out how to behave in a new kind of relationship is to approximate the new relationship to an existing template: often, in this case, to see a youth worker as a kind of teacher or social worker. However, the relationship will (and should) feel different from that. Young people regularly report that the youth work relationship is where they feel treated as an equal (Merton *et al.* 2004; Spence and Devanney 2006). The closest template to this is often that of a friend.

A friend?

The role approximation of friend can be appealing both to young people and to youth workers. However, it is not accurate and is misleading sometimes to the point of being dangerous. If, for example, youth workers count the young people they work with as friends and the young people see them in the same way, what are the rules? Do they drop into each others' houses and hang out together? Do they invite each other to parties? Do they go to the movies together, other than as a youth service activity? Do they go to the pub together? If so, do they buy each other alcohol? There is also the fact that youth workers are generally paid or otherwise mandated to be there. There is something a little wrong about being paid to be someone's friend.

As a generalisation, youth workers are not the friends of the young people with whom they work. They are their youth workers. It is no less a warm and caring relationship, but there are obligations and responsibilities that attach to the role of youth worker that do not attach to the role of friend, and vice versa. A youth worker's answer to a young person saying 'But I thought you were my friend!' should always be clear and unequivocal: 'I was never your friend: I am your youth worker.'

A second mum?

Another template for some workers is that of 'mum' (for some reason, the 'dad' approximation does not seem to be so common). This is an appealing, caring and nurturing role, and some of the young people with whom youth workers work may not have great relationships with their own mothers. It is easy for workers to be drawn into surrogate motherhood as a template for the relationship.

Some youth accommodation or residential services have worked with role descriptions of workers as 'house parents' or similar designations. Again, there is nothing wrong with that, and the way in which many care agencies are set up evokes short-term foster family models. However, the limitations and boundaries of these relationships need to be clear, including the way in which they differ from real parents. This does not necessarily need to be explained in explicit detail to young people, except when boundaries are being crossed or there are boundary mistakes being made. Generally, if youth workers are clear, act consistently within their role, and correct boundary crossings when they occur, young people will work out quite quickly how to find the complementary role.

Mother roles in a youth work context are not, in themselves, a bad thing. Many traditional societies actively organise multiple mothers within the culture, in recognition of this need. It is fine to have 'mum-type' workers as volunteers in youth agencies, and 'camp mum and dad' is a standard and rich tradition in residential or camping contexts. However, it is important to be careful in both the naming and explanation of such roles. The people in such positions are not youth workers. If they are youth workers, they should not be called 'mum' and 'dad'. The youth work relationship is a professional relationship, not a family one.

The professional relationship

The general consensus is that dual relationships should be avoided where possible, because it is difficult to avoid *conflicts of interest*: that is, what you should be doing in one role conflicts with what you should be doing in the other (Corey *et al.* 2007). The point is that the youth work relationship, unlike friend or family or even workmate relationships, is a *professional* relationship.

This is not uncontroversial, as other contributions to this book indicate. However, there are strong reasons why intervention with vulnerable people has been disciplined by the traditions of professional practice. The professional relationship puts *extra responsibilities* on youth workers and other professionals, over and above what would be the case in other commercial or personal relationships. In a commercial relationship, I trust the other person with my possessions or perhaps my time. In a professional relationship, I entrust them with *myself*.

The literature on the professions is extensive, and there are a number of competing conceptions of what a profession is and what it means to be a professional (see Callahan 1988; Koehn 1994). It is important to clarify how I am using the term and what implications that has for dual or multiple relationships in youth work. The fact that a lot has been written about professions is not surprising. Of all the relationship paradigms in our society, the idea of the professional has been stolen, rationalised, abused, borrowed, distorted, vaunted and maligned. Occupations of all sorts from carpet cleaners to car salespeople to people who beat other people up for a living have sought the name of 'professional' for their trade. To say that someone is *not* a professional is no longer just a description, it is an insult both to their integrity and their competence. On the other side, a succession of sociologists and social commentators have pointed out exactly how corrupt the professions are, how they masquerade as something noble while acting as a vehicle for the greed of their members, and how they all support the status quo (see Illich *et al.* 1977).

This is not the place for an extended discussion of the nature of the professions (for more details see Chapter 1 and also Sercombe 2004). Suffice to say that the concept has perhaps been borrowed so much *because* true professionalism in the helping professions has a character about it in terms of service that is genuinely other-directed, even altruistic, of high quality, and frequently courageous beyond the normal call of duty (Hughes 1963). This is why people want to appropriate it. It is important to identify the core ideal or spirit of the professional against which our actual practice may be measured (Koehn 1994). Key features of the core ideal are: that 'profession' is a relational term; that codes, training and legal status are designed to protect the professional relationship (rather than constituting it); and that professionals have a commitment to service.

'Professional' is a relational term

The term 'professional' does not initially describe a state or a status, but a relationship (Koehn 1994; Martin 2002). It is a relational term, like 'parent' or 'partner'. As a parent must have a child, so there must also be, for a professional, a client. If there is no client, there is no professional (Koehn 1994). In the case of youth work, the dyad is youth worker/young person. In youth work we largely avoid the use of the term 'client', probably out of sensitivity to experiences of condescension or lack of respect in our previous professional encounters. Professional relationships are not always condescending or paternalistic, however. A successful business person would not feel inferior when they are described as a client by their lawyers or stockbrokers. The term itself is not inherently negative. For ease of reference I will continue to use the term 'client' in this discussion of professional relationships.

This relationship is intentionally limited (Bayles 1981). These limits are in place in order to create conditions of safety within which clients can make themselves vulnerable (Koehn 1994). Typically, this is through some sort of disclosure: they are able to tell someone about ugly, guilty, embarrassing, dangerous or broken aspects of themselves. The idea is that the opportunity for such disclosure can be the first step towards transformation. When commentators talk about the importance of trust, they are talking about the process by which a client makes the decision that it is safe to be vulnerable.

In youth work, the disclosure is often not verbal and the intervention is often not verbal either. Much of the transformation that we hope for happens without intensive behind-closed-doors talking, but in apparently casual interactions that nevertheless have a quality about them that takes young people somewhere they otherwise would not have been able to go. The great skill of youth workers lies precisely in the capacity to be transformative, to create possibilities for a different and more whole way of being, even in the light, playful and casual everyday. In fact, intensive behind-closed-doors talking is not a big proportion of most youth workers' working day, unless counselling is part of their job description. Often it is more a case of youth workers knowing that something is going on with a young person and the young people knowing that the youth worker knows. Workers then create a kind of space within which options, alternatives and different ways to be can emerge. Talking is important, but it does not mean that nothing has happened if the talk has not taken place.

The vulnerability is not down to any deficit in young people as such. Young people are emerging into adulthood and there is a transformation that is going on in the teenage years, a confirmation of the self and their position in the world, which does involve some risk. Social conditions of exclusion and poverty exacerbate the risk and distort what should be (and still is for many) an interesting, difficult, fun and celebrated process. Youth work creates spaces within which that can occur successfully, and walks alongside young people through the process of it happening. This understanding is, I think, critical. The youth work profession works to create a kind of space within which youth workers will meet a young person and work with them, regardless of who they are and where they have come from in order to create possibilities of transformation. It is a partnership within that space (May (1975) calls it a covenant) in which youth worker and young person work together to help clear barriers, repair damage and promote new ways of being. It does not always work, but it does work often enough.

Strategies to protect the professional relationship

Codes of ethics, professional associations, training and recognition in law – the usual characteristics of a profession – are essentially strategies designed to protect the inner and outer integrity of the circle of the professional relationship. In terms of the inner integrity, they are designed to ensure that the intimacy developed within that circle stays within its purpose: the healing, defence and transformation of the client. Sexual expression is excluded from the relationship because it exploits an intimacy which had a different pretext and which held a promise that it would be protected from the complications and mixed motives of sexual demand. Economic intimacies, such as gifts, inheritances or exchanges are similarly excluded.

In terms of the outer integrity, the practice of confidentiality makes sure that the safety of the professional relationship is not betrayed by exposure to the outside world – even to other professionals – without the explicit consent of the client. The classical professions have the right to confidentiality guaranteed (with some conditions) in law. Others, such as journalists, make an ethical commitment to keep confidences in spite of what the law might do. The principle of *duty of care* takes responsibility for ensuring that the relationship does not place the client in further jeopardy.

Contrary to the view expressed by many commentators (e.g. Bayles 1981), a profession is not constituted by features such as codes of ethics, professional associations and university training. The profession already exists. These strategies are put in place to protect and strengthen the professional commitment that is already made.

Commitment to service

The stance of the professional is, according to Koehn (1994), established by a kind of *pledge or commitment* to a client group to serve within some prescribed area of action: defence against accusation, repair of the body, healing of the mind or emotions, the cure of souls. Professionals profess that their purpose is to serve their clients. Again, she argues, expertise or training are secondary, a way of fulfilling the commitment a professional has already made: in the case of youth workers this is the commitment to young people. The commitment is not always made overtly, though it would not be a bad idea if it was. In some cases it is, such as the Hippocratic Oath that doctors used to take (and in some parts of the world, still do). In others, subscribing to a code of ethics or some other standard constitutes that kind of pledge or commitment.

The relationship is not a symmetrical relationship, but a relationship of service. It is in its nature other-directed. The professional is there to serve the client, not the other way round. Professional service certainly has its rewards, and some of them may come from clients, but the professional is not hard done by if they do not, and clients are not responsible for them. In particular, the professional relationship is not a commercial or contractual relationship, though contracts may sometimes be used within them (May 1975). Clients are not customers buying a service. The notion of 'service' that is integral to the traditional conception of the professions is primarily a verb, something we do, and not a noun, a product we deliver.

In some earlier conversations on this topic (Sercombe 1997, 2004), and incorporated into the Code of Ethics for Youth Work used extensively in Australia

(Youth Affairs Council of Western Australia 2003), this commitment to service has been defined for youth work as the commitment *to engage the young person as the primary client, in their social context*. Actual practices and settings can and do vary widely, but youth workers hold in common their commitment to give priority to the interests of young people and to work not only towards the transformation of the young person in their social context but also the transformation of that context. Where the interests of funding bodies, governments, sponsoring organisations, parents or communities conflict with those of young people, priority should be given to the interests of young people. Youth workers should never act against the interests of young people.

Conflicts of interest

These three features of the professional relationship are critical for youth work. In the informal contexts in which youth work occurs, youth workers need to be clear about the nature of their relationship, and especially the limits of that relationship. It is the limits of the relationship that define it, that create its quality, and that channel its energy. This is probably true of any relationship. What people will not do in a relationship is just as important as what they will do. Different kinds of relationships have different codes for that. In a marriage, for example, a person may get up in the middle of the night to meet their obligations to their partner, but generally they would not take on another partner, at least not without discussing it with their first partner. A psychologist would probably not get up in the night for a client (unless on call), but there is not a problem with having more than one client, even if none of them knows about the other. Youth workers need to know what the youth work relationship is about: what they are doing, and perhaps even more importantly, what they are not doing.

Differences in obligations are the core of the dual role problem. When a young person is relating to a worker, which relationship is in play, what limits are in force and what are the rules? If, for example, youth workers count the young people they work with as friends, and the young people see them in the same way, what are the rules?

Family relationships are even more fraught. If a young man in a youth project is the male worker's nephew, is the youth worker in a particular moment the young man's uncle or his youth worker? If the worker is clear about the difference, is the young person also clear? Does the young person feel free to ask the worker for money, for example? If the young person was not the worker's nephew, would the young person still be asking, and would the youth worker be giving? Does the young person's mother, the worker's sister, expect to be kept informed about what is happening for her son? What is the worker's obligation to her, as his sister, versus his obligation as a professional to keep matters confidential?

In his role as a youth worker, Jim knows that his nephew, Chris, is using drugs. He also knows that his sister, Chris's mother, does not know. Should Jim tell? If he does not, and something bad happens to Chris – say, he is arrested for possession of drugs or has an accident – and it comes out that Jim knew he was using, how is his sister going to feel about that? How is Jim's reputation going to be in his family? His obligation as a youth worker is clear: he should keep confidences. The information belongs to the young person and it is not Jim's to hand around. Jim's obligations as an uncle and a brother are also quite clear: he should probably pass on information that Chris's parents need in order to care for their son effectively, especially if he is at immediate risk.

Should Jim tell Chris's mother about his drug use or not?

Unfortunately, in this instance, the two sets of obligations directly contradict each other. If Chris, the young person, tells Jim something as his youth worker, he has an absolute right to expect that confidence to be kept, and to feel betrayed if Jim were to break that confidence and tell his mother, regardless of the cultural context. If some damage occurred to Chris because the worker broke confidence (for example, if his mother threw him out) he would be well within his rights to sue for professional malpractice.

Good communication is essential in cases like this. If Jim's sister in the above example knows that he cannot pass on information about Chris that he has gained in the youth work relationship, no matter what the circumstances (short of the normal limits to confidentiality), and everyone involved can endorse that stance, then harm might be avoided if and when an actual situation arises. And Jim's client, his nephew Chris, knows what he can trust Jim for and what he cannot.

Equity

There is also a potential problem of equity, another principle covered in most codes of ethics. Do the young people who have a connection to a youth worker get more access to the worker and the services they provide than those who do not?

A youth work project is funded to deliver services in a country town. The youth worker was born and raised in the town and has a reasonable spread of personal connections with young people based on his own history. This is a ready-made constituency and the young people who have a personal or family connection to the youth worker get a very fine service indeed, with lots of money spent on them and camps every other weekend. However, most young people in the town do not even know that the youth service exists. The youth worker is busy enough without going outside their natural circle. Is this a problem?

The ethical principle, in this case, is that access to youth work services should be equitable – that is, distributed fairly according to need. Certainly, the youth worker often cannot work with every young person in the town, and some filters on participation will always be in place. However, if the main filter is about whether a young person is a friend or relative of the youth worker, it may mean that many young people with a more urgent claim for support may be denied a service. This is inequitable – and wrong.

Youth work versus personal business

There is also the problem of mixing up the kind of business in which youth workers are engaged. On the surface, the sorts of things youth workers do with young people can look very much like the kinds of activities they might do with their own friends: hanging out, drinking coffee, playing pool, going camping, going to amusement parks or sailing or riding horses. This might be part of an engagement strategy, by which young people are introduced to the possibilities that a professional relationship might offer, or it might be a youth work strategy about seeing what happens to young people's sense of possibility when they do things that are outside their normal experience. However, this may also create some problems.

Case study 5.3

A youth worker has risen through the ranks, from being a young person who came to the club, through a period as a volunteer, to now being the main person around for the daytime shift. Over time, the clientele of the daytime shift has changed, and now comprises a small group of mostly young men in their late teens and early twenties who also happen to be acquaintances of the youth worker. How can this issue be tackled?

In this case, there seems to be little difference between this young man hanging out with his mates as a mate, and hanging out with his mates as a youth worker, except that he gets paid for the latter (or rather, the taxpayer is paying for him and his recreation and that of his friends). One could speculate about what would happen to the funding for his project, and to the resources then available for young people in general, if this was discovered and became public. Again, the service has an obligation to be equitable, and in this case it is unlikely that all eligible young people would feel free to participate. The youth service needs to rethink the daytime programme and do some promotion, and probably consider moving staff around.

Buying and selling

A different kind of problem arises in commercial relationships with young people: buying and selling goods in particular. Whatever the advantages to both parties, the practice of selling goods to young people or buying from them is fraught with risks about the origin of the goods, disputes over payment, second thoughts about the fairness of the price, faulty goods or dissatisfaction with them – all of which could jeopardise the youth work relationship. If this is damaged or lost, it could mean that a young person now does not have access to a youth work service, because the youth work relationship has not been protected.

Avoiding dual role problems, or managing them

Given all the problems engendered by dual relationships, it is not surprising that the consensus across the professions is that dual relationships are to be avoided if at all possible (Corey *et al.* 2007). So if a youth worker happens to run across a young person with whom he works down at the pub, the worker smiles and says

'Hi' and turns back to his own group of friends. The worker does not join them and buy them a drink and move on to the nightclub with them when the pub closes. If the worker does not have any friends other than the young people, he needs help.

If the dual relationship cannot be avoided, strategies must be put in place to keep the relationships separate, and the separate roles clear, distinct and quarantined from each other. The following guidelines comprise some suggestions to help workers in this position.

Some guidelines for youth workers

1   Be clear about your role: about who and what you are as a youth worker and what your obligations are under your professional role and in your other roles. In this way you can identify where potential conflicts might arise. This is why it is absolutely essential that people have a clear notion of what a youth worker is, who they are as a youth worker, and what this entails ethically.

2   Be open and transparent with your peers about the potential for role conflict. In this way you can hold each other accountable, and catch role conflict when it happens. People are not generally good at watching over their own desires, and the potential for rationalisation and self-deception is considerable. In every case of role conflict, your supervisor should be notified of the potential for conflict of interest. This is yet another situation where routine professional supervision is important. If you are reluctant to tell your supervisor, it may be a sign that something is not quite right.

3   Wherever possible, do not work alone with a young person. Teamwork can dilute and offset dangers that exist in role confusion, and can help keep you in your youth worker role and accountable to that role.

4   Communicate clearly with the young person and with other stakeholders about the dual role and what your different roles require of you.

5   If role conflict is common or unavoidable within your field of practice, as it is in small towns, in situations where the practice is to promote young people into youth work roles, and in relationship-defined communities such as Aboriginal communities, codes of practice should be written into policy and procedures manuals so that everyone is clear and practitioners are not always having to work it out individually. Training and professional development is critical in these settings.

6   The onus of responsibility for the consequences of dual relationships, according to Corey *et al.* (2007), rests with the professional. If you enter into a dual relationship, it is up to you as the youth worker, not the young person, to manage the complexities involved.

7   Some people are good at quarantining different roles, at compartmentalising different kinds of relationships in their heads. Some are not. If you cannot

maintain a clear and distinct professional role with a young person because of a dual relationships problem, you may need to withdraw from that relationship and facilitate support for the young person with someone else. If dual relationships are unavoidable in the situation in which you work, you may need to find another job.

Conclusion

The notion of the professional role as intentionally limited is not one that has universal acceptance; nor is the idea that the youth work relationship is a professional relationship. Some practitioners would argue that the power of the youth work relationship is precisely the unlimited, unconditional support that is offered to a young person in crisis, the kind of support that a parent or brother or sister would give, and that the role has to be open-ended in its giving if transformation is to occur. Others would argue that young people are part of communities and that they and their communities have to be engaged together to work out solutions to the problems that young people might have. In this case, regardless of what the young person may want, information needs to be given to families and to the wider community to enable them to intervene where needed and indeed to change themselves where that is required.

This is a wider debate that we do not have the scope to enter into here. But there are good reasons why the professional tradition, with its understanding of the professional relationship as limited and privileged, has such a significant influence in practices that involve the proper and safe care of vulnerable people. The avoidance of dual relationships is one practice that protects the professional relationship, and avoids conflicts and complications that might compromise it. Sometimes this is possible, and sometimes it is not. In certain sections of the youth work field, complete avoidance of dual relationships is impossible, and the maintenance of integrity and clarity in the face of multiple relationships can be hard. I have been involved in dual relationships myself, both as a client and as a professional, sometimes by necessity, sometimes by choice. Sometimes they have worked well, and we have been able to preserve both roles successfully, and even to enrich them. Sometimes that has not happened, and one role has contaminated the other to the detriment of both. The writing of this chapter is in no small measure a response to my own mistakes.

None of the professions absolutely prohibits dual relationships (except sexual ones) – not only because they cannot always be avoided, but because they are not always unhelpful, and do not always result in exploitation of the client or in vicious conflicts of interest. Many codes of ethics, however, advise caution and a heightened attention to supervision and accountability when dual roles are involved (Corey *et al.* 2007). This is especially so for youth workers, because this way of working tends to promote relationships in which the power differences are kept in the background, the communication style feels like a friendship, and the professional encounter is not neatly circumscribed in time and space. Under these circumstances, awareness, debate, guidance and the pursuit of clarity about good practice are essential for the safety and integrity both of youth workers and young people.

Questions for reflection and discussion

1   When young people who have been youth service participants move into youth worker roles, should there be a clear rite of passage to indicate that they are no longer clients of the service but youth workers? How might this be achieved?

2   If a youth worker receives a message on her social networking site from a young person asking to be her friend, should she accept? If she does, what access do young people have to pictures or information about her private life?

3   In small communities, is a person employed as a youth worker ever *not* the youth worker? If most of their relationships are dual relationships to some extent, how can potential ethical conflicts be managed?

Recommended reading

Corey, G., Corey, M. and Callanan, P. (2007) *Issues and Ethics in the Helping Professions*, Belmont: Thomson. While this text aims for a broad reach of helping professions, it is principally concerned with counselling. Nevertheless, its treatment of the dual relationships problem is thorough and easily adaptable to youth work settings.

Koehn, D. (1994) *The Ground of Professional Ethics*, London: Routledge. Daryl Koehn's careful scholarly work forms the philosophical foundation to most of the perspectives in this chapter. She comes from a law background rather than youth work, but her material is highly applicable.

Sercombe, H. (2010) *Ethics in Youth Work*, London: Sage. This new book about youth work ethics explores the ethical implications of youth work understanding itself as a profession. The chapter on boundaries extends this discussion, and the chapter on sexuality also explores that particular dual relationships problem in more detail.

References

Bayles, M. (1981) *Professional Ethics,* Belmont: Wadsworth Publishing.

Callahan, J.C. (ed.) (1988) *Ethical Issues in Professional Life,* New York: Oxford University Press.

Cook, A.F. and Hoas, H. (2001) 'Voices from the margins: a context for developing bioethics-related resources in rural areas', *American Journal of Bioethethics/ bioethics.net,* www.bioethics.net/journal/pdf/cook-hoas.pdf (accessed May 2009).

Corey, G., Corey, M. and Callanan, P. (2007) *Issues and Ethics in the Helping Professions,* Belmont: Thomson.

Gottlieb, M.C. (1993) 'Avoiding exploitive dual relationships: a decision-making model', *Psychotherapy,* 30: 41–48.

Hughes, E. (1963) 'Professions', *Daedalus,* 92: 655–668.

Illich, I., Zola, I.K., McKnight, J., Caplan, J. and Shaiken, H. (1977) *Disabling Professions,* New York: Marion Boyars.

Koehn, D. (1994) *The Ground of Professional Ethics,* London: Routledge.

Martin, L. (2002) *The Invisible Table: Perspectives on Youth and Youthwork in New Zealand,* Wellington: Dunmore Press.

May, W. (1975) 'Code and covenant or philanthropy and contract', *Hastings Center Report,* 5: 29–38.

Merton, B., Payne, M. and Smith, D. (2004) *An Evaluation of the Impact of Youth Work in England,* Nottingham: Department for Education and Skills/De Montfort University, Youth Affairs Unit.

Schank, J.A. and Skovholt, T.M. (1997) 'Dual-relationship dilemmas of rural and small-community psychologists', *Professional Psychology: Research and Practice,* 28: 44–49.

Sercombe, H. (1997) 'The youth work contract: professionalism and ethics', *Youth Studies Australia,* 16: 17–21.

Sercombe, H. (2004) 'Disciplining youth work', *Commonwealth Youth and Development,* 2: 64–80.

Sercombe, H. (2006) 'Going bush: youth work in rural settings', *Youth Studies Australia,* 25: 9–16.

Spence, J. and Devanney, C. (2006) *Youth Work: Voices of Practice,* Leicester: The National Youth Agency.

Younggren, J.N. (2003) 'Ethical decision-making and dual relationships', www. kspope.com/dual/younggren.php#copy (accessed January 2009).

Youth Affairs Council of Western Australia (2003) *A Code of Ethics for Youth Work,* www.yacwa.org.au/files/Code%20of%20Ethics%20Booklet.pdf (accessed July 2008).

Youth workers as moral philosophers

Developing right thinking and mindfulness

Kerry Young

Introduction

This chapter proposes and then explores the idea that youth work is an exercise in moral philosophy and that youth workers support this process through engaging with young people in critical dialogue based on right thinking and mindfulness. This is an important contribution to young people's personal and social development because young people, like all people, want to live the life of good human beings.

Different people have different ideas about what it means to be a 'good' person. Yet most people for most of the time like to think of themselves as good, in whatever way they conceptualise 'good'; or, at the very least, they do not like to think of themselves as bad, in whatever way they conceptualise bad. That is my first premise. My second premise is that this matters. It matters to us how we see ourselves and how we are seen by others. If it did not matter we would spend less time and effort explaining, rationalising and justifying who we are and what we do. We would be happy that taking something which (strictly speaking) does not belong to us makes us a thief, and that giving a deliberately misleading account of events makes us a liar. However, generally we are not happy with such descriptions. We are not happy because while many of us may, on occasion, take something that (strictly speaking) does not belong to us (for example, making a private phone call from work) few of us would call that stealing or would want to be described as a thief as a result. Furthermore, while stealing may describe an action, being a thief describes the kinds of people we are. This is difficult for us given that, for the most part, we are people who continually seek to convince ourselves (and others) of the justifiable reasons for our behaviour, and the mitigating factors or extenuating circumstances of our actions – be they unwholesome thoughts or unkind deeds. In short, we want to make who we are and what we do acceptable. We prefer to see ourselves as good people – and if not good, then certainly not bad. However, if goodness is to be more than an exercise in mental gymnastics, then human beings must commit themselves to actually being good, or at least trying to be, in terms that are meaningful to them.

In *The Art of Youth Work* (Young 2006) I argued that youth work is an exercise in moral philosophy that enables and supports young people to examine what they consider to be 'good or bad', 'right or wrong', 'desirable or undesirable' in relation to self and others. I argued that this represents the fundamental purpose of youth work, since youth work engages with young people precisely at that moment in their lives when they are beginning to ask 'Who am I?' and 'What sort of person am I?' These questions of identity are inextricably bound to personal values about good and bad, right and wrong as well as broader social concerns about 'How am I, and how are we, to live?' Consequently, youth work's commitment to young people's personal and social development may be understood in terms of:

- Personal development: the development of *the person* – their sense of self, identity and personal values.
- Social development: the development of young people as *social beings* who recognise that their values encapsulate, following Rokeach's (1973: 5) definition, the 'modes of conduct' (for example, telling the truth) and 'states of existence' (for example, justice) they consider to be both personally and socially preferable. This is akin to Kant's categorical imperative that people should 'act upon a maxim that can also hold as a universal law' (Kant 1991: 51). In other words, whatever we do or however we behave, we would also hold that others do the same – the ethic of reciprocity that the Christians call the 'Golden Rule': Do unto others as you would have them do unto you.

I described the 'art of youth work' as the ability of youth workers to make and sustain relationships with young people that provide the environment and opportunities for such moral philosophising through reflective conversations that help young people to explore their values, deliberate on the principles of their own moral judgements and make informed decisions and reasoned choices that can be sustained through committed action – not as an exercise to inculcate particular values or virtues, but rather to support young people to find their own truth about what matters to them, and what values underpin how *they* want to live and how they think *we should all* live. In engaging in this process of moral philosophising, young people develop their skills in critical thinking and rational judgement as they reflect upon and learn from their experience, and make sense of themselves, their lives and their world.

The rest of this chapter develops and builds on these ideas – considering how youth workers can help young people learn to be good and why it matters. In so doing, it explores:

- how youth workers can use critical dialogue, including the Socratic method, as an approach to engaging young people in conversations about the nature of 'goodness' and how to be 'good';
- the importance of right thinking and mindfulness as a foundation for critical dialogue;
- the qualities needed by youth workers in developing a mindfulness-based approach to their work with young people.

Learning to be good

Confucius (1979: 12) believed that 'the only worthwhile thing a man [*sic*] can do is to become as good a man as possible'. Yet what does it mean to be a good man or a good human being? For Aristotle, human beings, like all things, have a goal or function to perform. Like a flautist, whose goal or function is to play the flute and do so as well as possible, so too is the goal of human beings to do things that are distinctly human and do them as well as possible. For Aristotle, what distinguishes human beings from other animals is the capacity to be rational; therefore, distinctly human activities are rational activities. According to Aristotle (1987: 309): 'It is perfectly clear that it is the rational part of man [*sic*] which is the man himself, and that it is the virtuous man who feels the most affection for this part.' As Van Hooft (2006: 51) comments:

> So the fulfilment of the functions of being a human being, or being good at being a human being, consists in the exercise of rationality in actions that are rational. Aristotle refers to the rational activity that will make us happy as virtuous activity. We shall be happy, he says, when we act in accordance with virtue and we shall be most happy when we act in accordance with the highest form of virtue.

My intention is not to suggest a particular set of virtues that ought to be developed by young people, but rather to advocate a purpose for youth work in supporting young people to develop the kind of rational activity in thinking and action that leads to a virtuous life – that is, the virtuous life of a good (and happy) human being. I draw a distinction between the term 'virtues' which refers to *particular* moral qualities such as wisdom, courage, benevolence, compassion or trustworthiness; in contrast with 'virtue' meaning an overall disposition of character, which helps to determine what one will want to do in particular circumstances (Williams 1993: 9). Acting in accordance with virtue therefore requires that a person will choose to act in certain ways based on a disposition towards certain ideals or ethical principles. As such, the practice of virtue requires the ability to deliberate and make rational judgements. We are able to achieve this because a part of the human condition, according to Aristotle, is the ability to 'think about what we do, to plan our actions, to be strategic in our approach to our needs and to review the effectiveness of what we have done' (Van Hooft 2006: 54).

However, virtue is not only about thinking. It is also about action, for as Aristotle (1987: 351) commented: 'It is not enough to know the nature of virtue; we must endeavour to possess it, and to exercise it, and to use whatever other means are necessary for becoming good.' Indeed, a person acquires virtue by doing virtuous acts: 'It is by doing just acts that we become just, by doing temperate acts that we become temperate, by doing courageous acts that we become courageous' (Aristotle 1987: 43). There are, therefore, according to Preston (1993), two basic issues in relation to virtue: how to find right action in particular circumstances; and how to act from right motive.

Finding right action

Central to 'finding right action' is the ability to make reasoned choices, and yet, as Barrow (1975: 21) observed:

> No doubt for many of us, much of the time, the reasons that lie behind our actions are muddled, insufficiently worked out or only vaguely formulated in our minds. Nonetheless we choose to act in some ways rather than others and our choices are based on reason – for to make a choice is precisely to opt for one thing rather than another for some kind of reason.

Finding right action therefore requires the individual, first, to accept that she or he has choices, however limited or constrained; second, to discern those choices honestly and realistically; and third, to make decisions based on reasoned and rational judgement.

Acting from right motive

Acting from right motive requires that decision-making attends to feelings as well as thought, for, as David Hume argued, morality 'must be rooted in our feelings since morality moves us to action, and reason alone can never do so' (quoted in Schneewind 1993: 150). We must act with our heart as well as our head. Yet what is this heart?

Mencius (1970: 82) postulated that all people are born with an 'original heart' containing four incipient tendencies in 'germ' or seed form, which may be summarised as:

- compassion, the germ of benevolence;
- a sense of shame, the germ of dutifulness;

- courtesy and modesty, the germ of observance of the rites;
- right and wrong, the germ of wisdom.

The purpose of the heart is to think, and it is this, according to Mencius, which distinguishes human beings from animals. Yet the 'original heart' must be cared for, nurtured and cultivated in order to grow to full maturity. Therefore, through our own endeavour, human beings can perfect our own moral characters, building on whatever we have inherited whether from our 'original heart', family or community. For while people may inherit certain moral principles, they can none the less, through rational enquiry, devise their own solutions to the situations they encounter in ways that reform their own moral outlook (Dewey 1961).

In so doing, people make choices, since virtue is not simply a set of rules to be followed. Virtue requires thinking, reflection, the exercise of practical reason. We weigh one value against another – not simply in choosing whether to steal or not to steal, or to lie or not to lie – but in the more complex weighing of one 'good' (e.g. loyalty) against another 'good' (e.g. justice). We must choose to 'do the right thing' even if we risk appearing stupid or naïve to our associates; or even if doing so is to our apparent disadvantage. We must decide if it is acceptable to 'do the wrong thing' to get what we want. In the process of such deliberations, we uncover the moral principles and ethical ideals that underpin our decision-making, and come to recognise the 'coherent system of precepts' (Williamson 1997) within which we operate. It is from this vantage point that we are then able to enquire into those principles and ideals and engage in a rational and deliberate process of shaping our moral character. For, as Parekh (1993: 65) argues, virtues are not simply motives for action, or moral qualities or skills that a person may possess. Virtues are about conduct and character; about rightness and goodness; about what we should do and how we should be: 'Virtues are a moral compass for mapping, ordering and finding one's bearings in life.'

My contention is that youth work enables and supports young people to uncover and create their 'moral compass' and fashion their moral character through:

- Engaging in 'moral enquiry' about what is 'good' and conducive to the life of a 'good human being' – the ability that Aristotle called the development of practical wisdom.
- Developing 'right thinking', as the groundwork that enables them to find right action in particular circumstances and to act from right motive.

Moral enquiry

> Morality is not a matter of seeking something apart from the self – it is simply the discovery of something within the self.
>
> (Nishida 1990: 145)

Moral enquiry involves reflection. It involves looking deeply into our experience and questioning ourselves about our own actions and motives, and the actions and motives of others. It involves considering the world from a broader perspective, not merely from our own self-interest. It is an educational process in the sense of being about learning; and a therapeutic process in the sense of seeking to have a positive effect on mind and body.

In the youth work context, it involves conversation – conversation that is educational in its purpose and intent, combined with a commitment to facilitate learning (Ord 2007:15). This is conversation that uses young people's own experiences in order to help them to develop their reflective behaviour. Such conversation inhabits the realm of both personal and social development, and is committed to 'education for liberation' in the sense that it enables and supports young people to:

> Reflect on themselves, their responsibilities, and their role in the [new] cultural climate – indeed to reflect on the very power of reflection. The resulting development of this power [being] an increased capacity for choice.
>
> (Freire 1976:16)

Critical dialogue and the Socratic method

So this enquiry and reflection is no idle or ordinary chat. It is a thoughtful and committed engagement in which young people are supported to:

- reflect on their experience (reflecting not only on what they think but also on how they feel);
- consider different views of the world;
- formulate general premises and principles, ideas or theories based on their observations of everyday life; and test them against the general principles, ideas and theories of others.

It is a critical dialogue, in the sense that people commit themselves to a mutual exploration in order to gain greater understanding and insight. Yet it is more than this; more than the identification and resolution of disagreement or uncertainty; more than a dispassionate exercise of the intellect. For to motivate people towards action, such dialogue must assume a transformational quality so that people are concerned not only with what they think about philosophical concepts and moral questions, but with how they feel and how they act. This cooperative activity in philosophising epitomises the Socratic method since 'central to Socratic philosophy is the moral agent, the human agent who has to think about how he or she is to live well with others in social harmony' (Saran and Neisser 2004: 4). Moreover, as Leal (2004: 123) suggests:

The main assumption behind a Socratic Dialogue, the philosophical bottom line, is that deep inside ourselves we have knowledge about the most important things which should concern human beings, namely how we ought to live.

Socratic dialogue is envisaged, therefore, not as a question-and-answer interrogation designed to uncover universal truths but as a conversation in which participants (in this case young people) are supported to come to know what they think, believe and feel, through a conversation that involves mutual respect and freedom of thinking. In other words, it is an exercise in practical reasoning and rational judgement by autonomous human beings – that is, people capable of acting in accordance with reason and from their own free will, voluntarily as opposed to acting 'under compulsion or from ignorance' (Aristotle 1987: 66).

Saran and Neisser (2004: 3) describe Socratic dialogue as an activity in cooperative thinking where the basic aims are:

- To answer a philosophical question by seeking out the truth about the nature of concepts such as tolerance, freedom, justice and responsibility, and to endeavour to reach consensus – i.e. to reach a result or *outcome*.
- To engage in the cooperative activity of seeking answers to questions and to understand each other through the exploration of *concrete experiences*, volunteered by participants, one of which is usually chosen by the group for detailed analysis. In this way all are engaged in the *process*.
- To deepen individual *insights and understandings* as the dialogic process moves towards enabling participants to grasp the moral perplexities of the everyday world.
- To gain through dialogue greater clarity about what is and what is not in keeping with considered, thoughtful and reasonable conduct, thus enhancing self-confidence in our ability to reason and so shaping our *approach to life*.

Socratic dialogue is, therefore, 'the art of teaching not philosophy but philosophising, the art not of teaching about philosophers but of making philosophers' (Nelson 2004: 126). In the process, participants are encouraged to:

- Develop 'Socratic virtues' such as listening, openness, reflection, practical reasoning, patience, trusting one's doubts, suspending judgement.
- Examine the fundamental nature of philosophical questions and concepts.
- Reach consensus, not as an aim in itself, but as a means to deepen investigation and understanding.
- Weigh new insights in terms of their significance for their own lives.

(Society for the Furtherance of the Critical Philosophy 2009)

My view is that such an exercise in collective enquiry and critical dialogue can be undertaken by youth workers not only within a formalised group-based context, but also with any number of young people, including individuals, since what is required is not necessarily the structured group process typically associated with Socratic dialogue, but rather a willingness to participate, share experience, contribute honest thinking and commit to listening. As Leal (2004: 123) comments:

> The main thing is to listen, to listen to other people and to listen to yourself. And when you listen to others, it is not only to know whether they have understood you, but to know whether you have understood them. Only then will you enable them to listen to themselves . . . The Socratic work is a work of cooperation, a way of thinking together and growing together.

This cooperation, thinking and growing can be achieved with individual young people as positively and as meaningfully as with groups, provided that the youth worker is able to meet the demands of the Socratic method, which calls for 'tenacity, discipline, patience, humour and intelligence' (Leal 2004: 123).

Developing skills in Socratic and other forms of critical dialogue is important for youth workers not only because they need to develop their critical skills in reflective and deliberative processes (i.e. the moral philosophising through which they seek to support young people), but also because such skills are crucial to workers' own reflections, for example, in exploring the philosophical under-pinnings of their practice in terms of the assumptions, beliefs and values that underpin their work.

Right thinking

Such reflection requires 'right thinking' – that is, thinking based on perception that is free from ignorance and delusion. However, as Smart (1993: 125) comments, 'the kind of knowledge which replaces ignorance is not merely intellectual; it is a kind of knowledge involving experience and a kind of vision'. Nishida (1990) suggests that experience devoid of delusion is *pure* experience – experience 'just as it is without the least addition or deliberative discrimination'. According to Nishida (1990: 3):

> The true unity of consciousness is a pure and simple activity that comes forth of itself, unhindered by oneself; it is the original state of independent, self-sufficient consciousness . . . At this time our true personality expresses itself in its entirety. Personality therefore is not found in mere reason or desire, much less in unconscious impulses; like the inspiration of a genius, it is an infinite unifying power that functions directly and spontaneously from within each individual.

My suggestion is that youth work, in engaging young people in 'moral enquiry', must necessarily support them to develop 'right thinking' as the essential foundation of being able to find right action and to act from right motive.

The Zen Buddhist monk Thich Nhat Hanh (1999: 60–62) identifies four practices underpinning right thinking, which may be summarised as follows:

- *Are you sure?* – Wrong perceptions cause incorrect thinking. If there is a rope in your path and you perceive it as a snake, fear-based thinking will follow. The more erroneous your perception, the more incorrect your thinking will be. To develop right thinking you have to ask yourself this question: 'Are you sure?' again and again.
- *What am I doing?* – Asking yourself 'What am I doing?' will help you to stay in the present moment, thereby allowing you to be mindful and enabling you to be a resource for others.
- *Hello (habit energy)* – Our way of acting depends on our way of thinking, and our way of thinking tends to repeat old habits – even the ones that are unhelpful to us, and others. We need to recognise our habitual patterns of thinking and acting in order to diminish their power over us.
- *Mind of love* – Our 'mind of love' is our loving kindness and compassion. With loving kindness and compassion at the foundation of our thinking, everything we do or say will help others to be liberated.

Mindfulness

Recent developments in mindfulness-based stress reduction and cognitive therapy focus on the clinical applications of mindfulness for treating anxiety, stress, depression, chronic pain and illness (e.g. Centre for Mindfulness Research). Yet mindfulness has a long and distinguished history at the heart of Buddhist teachings where it is an everyday practice, a practice for life, which involves being in the present moment; being aware of what one is doing, saying, thinking and feeling in the present moment. Right mindfulness means being fully present, aware and attentive, and not being overwhelmed by impetuous or unwholesome actions or reactions. For Buddhists, there are four foundations of mindfulness which Hanh (1999) identifies as: mindfulness of the body; mindfulness of feeling; mindfulness of thought; and mindfulness of mind objects (knowing whether the thought is wholesome or unwholesome). However, according to Hanh (2008: 22):

> Just returning to the present moment does not necessarily mean that I am able to dwell there with stability and freedom. I can be carried away by what is happening and lose myself . . . Practicing mindfulness, I can recognise what is happening in the present without grasping or aversion. I can practice mere recognition of what is going on within me and around me. This helps me to keep stability and freedom alive within myself.

A mindfulness-based approach to youth work offers young people the opportunity to learn how to take charge of themselves and their lives in the present moment, being aware of what they are doing, saying, thinking and feeling in that present moment – whether that is a moment of a lived experience or a moment of active reflection. For if youth work is, as I propose, an exercise in moral philosophising, it follows that youth workers must support young people to develop mindfulness as the foundation of their engagement in moral enquiry based on right thinking. By this means they help young people increasingly to:

• Recognise their habitual patterns, and the ways in which 'mindless acts' limit or are counter-productive to their lives and human flourishing.
• Grow their capacity to create a greater choice of 'being' physically, emotionally and spiritually.

The mindful practitioner

To be effective in this process of making philosophers out of young people, youth workers must commit themselves to reflecting continuously on their own values and the underlying ethical framework of their practice. In *The Art of Youth Work* (Young 2006: 99) I suggested that this should involve youth workers in 'disciplined discussion', which, following Kupperman (1983), consists of three essential components:

1 Serious discussion about values including getting people to see what it is like to live according to various value judgements.
2 Promotion of sensitivity to others and the consequences of one's actions.
3 Discussion of moral rules and principles (e.g. respect for persons).

However, it is more than this. It is more than the development of certain qualities (e.g. being fair, truthful or trustworthy) as a part of establishing the moral authority 'to ask questions about what might be good or bad' (Jeffs and Smith 2005: 98). It is a deeper question. As Moss (2007: 11) puts it:

> The age-old question 'who am I?' hangs tantalisingly over all our professional endeavours. It is the mirror into which we must daily gaze so that we do not allow our own prejudices to cloud our professional judgements. But it is also a much wider mirror – perhaps even a hall of mirrors – in which a kaleidoscope of images and responses bombards us with a multiplicity of responses with bewildering complexity.

That question 'who am I?' is the same question waiting for every young person who pauses to wonder about, or question the meaning and significance of their everyday life and experiences; who pauses to consider what is good or bad; or reflect on right and wrong. It is the same question which, I assert, lies at the heart of youth work.

Therefore, in order to develop an effective and credible practice, youth workers need to undertake that same journey I propose to be the youth work process. This involves:

- Learning how to find right action in particular circumstances; and how to act from right motive.
- Engaging in moral enquiry through reflection and conversation through a process of critical dialogue.
- Developing right thinking that is free from ignorance and delusion and involving the four practices: *Am I sure? What am I doing? Hello (habit energy); Mind of love.*
- Developing mindfulness as a practice for living life in the present moment – fully present, aware and attentive.

The practice of mindfulness offers youth workers a way to discover and nurture the true presence and real listening needed for *this* youth work; understanding youth work not as a set of skills or techniques, but as a state of being; shifting from 'doing mode' to 'being mode' with mindfulness as a way of 'paying attention with empathy, presence and deep listening' (Hick and Bien 2008: 5).

At its heart, mindfulness is a way of being with another person or persons. It is a way of 'cultivating, sustaining and integrating a way of paying attention to the ebb and flow of emotions, thoughts and perceptions within all human beings' (Hick and Bien 2008: 13). As Hanh (2006: 136) comments:

> Mindfulness is the best state of being for the mind. With mindfulness, our thinking and our bodily and verbal actions will go in the direction of healing and transforming.

Why it matters

It matters because, in our hearts, human beings want to be good. We want to think of ourselves as good; we want others to think of us as good; and we will construct a conception of goodness that allows us to be good – that allows us to believe that whatever we do is the right thing. This means that we will sometimes act from a belief that what we are doing is right, or sometimes we will choose to act out of fear, or duty, or obligation to others, or for self interest, or for the praise or rewards our actions might bring. We will make our actions (attitudes and beliefs) right in our own mind. We will offer explanations or excuses. On other occasions we will claim that we had no choice or that what we do or think is what everyone does or thinks. Sometimes we will deny that it matters. But it does. I have not yet met a person who, deep down inside, felt good about being a bad person. People who genuinely think of themselves as bad people generally feel bad about themselves. That is because ethics is practical. We want to be able to live our ethics. We want to be able to live in good faith with ourselves. We want to be authentic.

When we choose to live an ethical life based on mindfulness and right thinking that is free from ignorance and delusion; where we reflect on our own experiences and consider the world from a broader perspective; where we make positive choices and act accordingly; where through rational enquiry we discover and perfect our 'moral compass'; then we will have created a way of living that gives the rewards of a 'good reputation and an easy conscience' (Singer 1997: 227). And we will flourish not only in achieving our goals, but in living in peace with ourselves and with others.

All we need is 'an awareness of the power of imagination to shape our perception of virtue, and the power of courage to enable us to live virtuously' (Darling-Smith 1993: 13).

Conclusion

This chapter has explored the idea of what it means to conceive of youth workers taking on the role of moral philosophers in their relationships with young people. This conception of youth workers as moral philosophers focuses attention on the ways in which they help young people learn how to be good by engaging with them in critical dialogue about the fundamental nature of philosophical concepts and questions. Such dialogue is based within a framework of right thinking and mindfulness, which supports young people to conceptualise their own understanding of 'good' and what it means to be a 'good' person. In the process, young people develop the insights, dispositions and skills to perfect their own moral character.

Questions for reflection and discussion

1   What evidence can you give to support the argument that youth work is an exercise in moral philosophy?

2   What evidence can you give to contest the argument that youth work is an exercise in moral philosophy?

3   If youth work is an exercise in moral philosophy, how can youth workers develop the qualities needed to become effective moral philosophers?

Recommended reading

Hanh, N. (1991) *The Miracle of Mindfulness,* London: Rider & Co. This book explains the essential discipline of mindfulness and provides anecdotes and practical exercises to develop greater self-understanding and daily mindfulness.

Van Hooft, S. (2006) *Understanding Virtue Ethics*, Stocksfield: Acumen Publishing. This useful textbook provides an introduction to the subject charting the history of virtue ethics from Aristotle to Nietzche and considers moral issues such as abortion and euthanasia.

Young, K. (2006) *The Art of Youth Work,* 2nd edn, Lyme Regis: Russell House Publishing. This book explores the contribution that youth work makes to young people's lives and argues that youth work's distinctiveness lies in its purposeful engagement of young people in the process of moral philosophising about their values and personal and social identity.

References

Aristotle (1987 edition) *The Nicomachean Ethics*, trans. J. Welldon, Buffalo, NY: Promethus Books.

Barrow, R. (1975) *Moral Philosophy for Education*, London: Allen & Unwin.

Centre for Mindfulness Research, Bangor University, www.bangor.ac.uk/mindfulness/ (accessed July 2009).

Confucius (1979 edition) *The Analects*, trans. D.C. Lau, Harmondsworth: Penguin.

Darling-Smith, B. (ed.) (1993) *Can Virtue be Taught?*, Notre Dame: University of Notre Dame Press.

Dewey, J. (1961) *Democracy and Education: An Introduction to the Philosophy of Education*, New York: Macmillan.

Freire, P. (1976) *Education: The Practice of Freedom*, London: Writers and Readers Publishing Cooperative.

Hanh, N. (1999) *The Heart of the Buddha's Teachings*, New York: Broadway Books.

Hanh, N. (2006) *Understanding Our Mind*, Berkeley, CA: Parallax Press.

Hanh, N. (2008) *Touching The Earth: Guided Meditations for Mindfulness Practice*, Berkeley, CA: Parallax Press.

Hick, S. and Bien, T. (eds) (2008) *Mindfulness and the Therapeutic Relationship*, New York and London: Guilford Press.

Jeffs, T. and Smith, M. (2005) *Informal Education: Conversation, Democracy and Learning*, 3rd edn, Nottingham: Educational Heretics Press.

Kant, I. (1991 edition) *The Metaphysics of Morals*, trans. Mary Gregor, Cambridge: Cambridge University Press.

Kupperman, J. (1983) *The Foundations of Morality*, London: Allen & Unwin.

Leal, F. (2004) 'The Socratic Method: an introduction to the essay of Nelson', in R. Saran and B. Neisser (eds) *Enquiring Minds: Socratic Dialogue in Education*, Stoke on Trent: Trentham Books.

Mencius (1970 edition) *[The] Mencius*, trans. D.C. Lau, Harmondsworth: Penguin.

Moss, B. (2007) *Values*, Lyme Regis: Russell House Publishing.

Nelson, L. (2004) 'The Socratic Method', in R. Saran and B. Neisser (eds) *Enquiring Minds: Socratic Dialogue in Education*, Stoke on Trent: Trentham Books.

Nishida, K. (1990) *An Inquiry into the Good*, trans. M. Abe and C. Ives, New Haven, CT, and London: Yale University Press.

Ord, J. (2007) *Youth Work Process, Product and Practice: Creating an Authentic Curriculum in Work with Young People*, Lyme Regis: Russell House Publishing.

Parekh, B. (1993) 'Bentham's theory of virtue', in B. Darling-Smith (ed.) *Can Virtue be Taught?*, Notre Dame: University of Notre Dame Press.

Preston, R. (1993) 'Christian ethics', in P. Singer (ed.) *A Companion to Ethics*, Oxford: Blackwell.

Rokeach, M. (1973) *The Nature of Human Values*, New York: Free Press.

Saran, R. and Neisser, B. (eds) (2004) *Enquiring Minds: Socratic Dialogue in Education*, Stoke on Trent: Trentham Books.

Schneewind, J. (1993) 'Modern moral philosophy', in P. Singer (ed.) *A Companion to Ethics*, Oxford: Blackwell.

Singer, P. (1997) *How Are We to Live? Ethics in an Age of Self-interest*, Oxford: Oxford University Press.

Smart, N. (1993) 'Clarity and imagination as Buddhist means to virtue', in B. Darling-Smith (ed.) *Can Virtue be Taught?*, Notre Dame: University of Notre Dame Press.

Society for the Furtherance of the Critical Philosophy, 'The Socratic Method', www.sfcp.org.uk/socratic_dialogue.htm (accessed July 2009).

Van Hooft, S. (2006) *Understanding Virtue Ethics*, Stocksfield: Acumen Publishing.

Williams, B. (1993) *Ethics and the Limits of Philosophy*, Hammersmith: Fontana Press.

Williamson, B. (1997) 'Moral learning: a lifelong task', in R. Smith and P. Standish (eds) *Teaching Right And Wrong: Moral Education in the Balance*, Stoke on Trent: Trentham Books.

Young, K. (2006) *The Art of Youth Work,* 2nd edn, Lyme Regis: Russell House Publishing.

7 Youth workers as controllers

Issues of method and purpose

Tony Jeffs and Sarah Banks

Introduction

Most commentators seem to agree that an agenda of control has become more explicit and more dominant within youth work in recent years (Davies 2008, 2009; de St Croix 2008). As one youth worker notes:

> It seems there is a general perception from people outside our discipline that youth workers are there to make young people conform, behave or toe the line. Of course, this has never been the purpose of youth work.
>
> (Jolly 2009: 9)

However, there is an ongoing debate about whether youth workers should embrace this control agenda as providing a socially recognised and valued rationale for the work, or whether it runs contrary to the values of youth work and corrupts its essential nature. In order to explore the issues involved in this debate more fully we will look at what is meant by 'control' in youth work.

'Youth workers as controllers' can have several different meanings. Recent debates about control in youth work have predominately focused around whether or not control, in the sense of diverting or preventing young people from pursuing activities considered harmful, should be regarded, and indeed promoted, as a core purpose of the work. There are some who argue strongly that youth work can make a big impact in this area and should not be shy about accepting funding explicitly for such targeted work and demonstrating its impact (France and Wiles 1996; 1997; Ord 2009; Smith and Paylor 1997). Others argue against such a position, claiming it is incompatible with an educational purpose for the work; it threatens the voluntary and universal nature of youth provision; marginalises those not regarded as problematic; works to an externally defined agenda rather than a local analysis of young people's needs; and undermines the service ideals of youth work (Jeffs 2004; Jeffs and Smith 1994, 1996, 2008).

There is another sense in which youth workers might be regarded as controllers, which reflects debates of the 1970s and 1980s about social control in welfare work (Corrigan and Leonard 1978; Langan and Lee 1989; see also de St Croix 2009). This position would acknowledge that the core purpose of the work is education, but would argue that even education is or can be controlling; that the purpose of education is in fact to socialise young people to fit into society and accept its norms. Although this brand of 'radical pessimism' has less purchase today, it is worth revisiting briefly to test its relevance to current debates.

The third sense of youth workers as controllers relates to methods and styles of practice, rather than purpose. If we regard the first two senses as 'practice for control', then this third is about 'control in practice'. This is less talked about today than in the past – having connotations of discipline, autocratic leadership, rules and punishment. Yet some degree of control on the part of youth workers is essential in order to create an appropriate learning environment, promote equality of opportunity and ensure the safety and well-being of young people. It is around this issue that many of the biggest day-to-day ethical dilemmas arise for workers: for example, how much influence or control should they exert without compromising the freedom and responsibility of the young people?

In order to shed light on this topic of youth workers as controllers we will begin by exploring control in practice, moving on to look at practice for control through education and through prevention/diversion.

Control in practice

Early practitioners generally held control and good discipline to be a, if not the, key to effective youth work. As one text warned novices:

> firm discipline is absolutely essential. More well-meant efforts for lads have failed through lack of ability to maintain good discipline than from any other cause.
>
> (Bickerdike 1926: 16)

Yet youth workers also recognised the dangers of excessive discipline and were concerned to differentiate youth clubs and youth workers from schools and teachers (Jephcott 1942; Russell and Russell 1932; Secretan 1931). Most schools were then, as they are today, obsessed with order and centralised management. As the following account of schooling in the late nineteenth century demonstrates, control was the prime task of the teacher, fuelling repeated admonition:

> Such phrases as 'Don't talk', 'Don't fidget', 'Don't worry', 'Don't ask questions', 'Don't make a noise', 'Don't make a mess', 'Don't do this thing', 'Don't do that thing', are ever falling from [the teacher's] lips. And they are

supplemented with such positive instructions as: 'Sit still', 'Stand on the form', 'Hold yourself up', 'Hands behind backs', 'Hands on heads', 'Eyes on the blackboard'.

(Davin 1996: 122)

Ultimately such instructions were enforced by recourse to the strap, slap and cane. Schools, especially those provided for the poor, were generally violent, dismal, boring places where attendance was often only secured by threats of legal action against parents and the incarceration of persistent truants (Hurt 1979). Within such an environment uniformity rather than creativity became the more desirable attribute since the latter, like imagination, was 'inconvenient to the teacher' (Russell 1932: 95).

Schools remain obsessed with order and conformity to rules and regulations rather than creativity and the intellectual development of students and staff. Control is now increasingly imposed via intensive surveillance, contracts, expulsion, suspension and 'whole school policies'. With regard to the first of these, in a growing number of schools not only are corridors, toilets and playgrounds monitored by cameras, but also classrooms during lessons (Shepherd 2009). The instigators of these practices tend to justify them in terms of promoting safety and good conduct (this might be expressed in terms of utilitarian ethical principles about preventing harm and promoting human welfare). On the other hand, it could be argued that such practices are intrusive and compromise the rights of staff and students to reasonable privacy. In considering whether such policies and practices are ethically warranted, we might draw on Rawls's (1951, 1999) method of ethical deliberation known as 'reflective equilibrium'. According to Rawls (1999: 19): 'Justification is a matter of the mutual support of many considerations, of everything fitting together into one coherent view', in contrast to justification by reference to a single principle or theory. The method tries to produce coherence between considered moral judgements or intuitions, moral principles, and relevant background theories. If we consider carefully the nature of the surveillance process (involving invasion of privacy and a lack of interpersonal trust), it is difficult to envisage that a youth worker would wish to encourage the acceptability of similar behaviour among young people – which might include evesdropping, spying and intruding upon private conversations. These practices of surveillance also ensure that in these classrooms and schools opportunities for honest, open and critical dialogue and debate are curtailed. Within such instutions it could be argued that it would be ethically unacceptable to engage in any but the most superficial of conversations with young people, as these would be recorded. This is an extreme but not unusual example of how the actions of adults designed to control and manage young people serve to make it difficult, if not impossible, for youth work, counselling or guidance in any meaningful sense to take place.

Compulsion, except briefly during the war years of 1939 to 1945, was never an option for youth work until recently. Youth workers knew from the onset that to make an impact meant cultivating ways of working which distanced them from school-teachers. According to Hannah More, possibly the first modern youth worker, this entailed learning to teach not by dull rote but by dialogue 'through animated conversation and lively discussion' (quoted in Collingwood and Collingwood 1990: 106). Baden-Powell also stressed the need to offer radically different approaches to those employed by schools in order to hold the allegiance of young people. He told his followers to be prepared to 'use as bait the food the fish likes . . . to hold out something that really attracts and interests them' (Baden-Powell 1908: 271). Youth workers in particular looked to group work (the Scouts and Guides called it the 'Patrol System') rather than classroom instruction as the means 'to develop people' (Kingman and Sidman 1935: 19). They placed substantial emphasis on the need to foster friendship between the adults and young people, self-discipline rather than imposed order, activities rather than passive instruction. Consequently youth work acquired a distinctive vocabulary which then, and now, helps distinguish it from school-based education. Leaders or workers and not teachers organised the learning; sessions and not periods or classes divided up the time; and participants were members, even clients, never students or pupils. Nevertheless, according to Baden-Powell (1908: 272) it was still important that 'discipline and good order should be kept inside the room, and neatness insisted on'.

Contemporary literature largely eschews the topic of club and centre discipline. Managers similarly refrain from issuing the sort of instructions Baden-Powell and his ilk handed down to a previous generation of workers. Nowadays the texts place disproportionate emphasis upon the management and discipline of workers, yet barely consider the question of discipline within the youth work setting (Ford *et al.* 2002; Robertson 2005; Sapin 2009). Yet although the topic is less openly discussed, contemporary workers cannot evade it; indeed, it is a point of discussion frequently raised in conversations among workers. Like progressive educators in the school sector, youth workers must continually wrestle with the problem of unearthing ways of managing and controlling the learning experience without resorting to harsh and inappropriate stratagems as well as discover approaches whereby neither subject nor teacher dominate yet enable learning to take place.

Workers of a previous generation had an intuitive belief that:

> collective discipline fails to develop the individual and as a result fails to bring forward the right kind of leader. It produces the drill-sergeant type as opposed to the imaginative Scoutmaster.
>
> (Phillips quoted in Gate 1933: 52)

This was a view which seemed to be confirmed by highly influential 'scientific' research undertaken by Lewin and his associates in the 1930s (Lewin *et al.* 1939). This contrasted with the impact of what they termed the autocratic, democratic and laissez-faire styles of leadership within boys' club settings. Their results strongly suggested that autocracy was generally accompanied either by rebellion or by submission on the part of the boys. It was highly productive when the autocratic leader was present, but destructive behaviour was common in the leader's absence. Democratic leadership was, they argued, more 'task-orientated, cooperative . . . friendly' (ibid.: 278), encouraging independent behaviour especially when the leader was not in attendance. Laissez-faire leadership did least for productivity, and was often accompanied by intra-group hostility. In almost every case the democratic style was preferred by the group. However, that is not to say the democratic style is appropriate in all situations, nor should it be assumed that a democratic worker never uses formal methods. Libertarian and progressive educators have always found it necessary to adopt formal methods to teach certain subjects (Shotton 1993), just as youth workers and informal educators must do so when working with young people in 'dangerous' settings such as canoeing or horse riding. Inevitably a problem regarding what is 'dangerous' arises, not least because the catagorisation of what is socially defined as being dangerous changes over time. Activities and behaviours so categorised have significantly expanded in recent years (Furedi 1997). As this has occurred, so the capacity of youth workers to allow young people the freedom to choose what to do and to act spontaneously has been curtailed. Very little, it seems, can now be done with young people without first obtaining parental consent and workers completing a 'risk assessment'. This discourages workers from being pro-active and encourages a safety-first or 'jobsworth' approach to the work as the need to control risk and eliminate the dangerous translates into a greater need to manage and control the young people.

However great the desire to foster imagination and teach via 'novelty, excitement, fun, a chance to explore new things' (Jephcott 1942: 67), youth workers have to exercise a measure of control over the learning experience. They have to temper their optimism that somehow the innate curiosity of young people will lead them naturally towards learning things that are of educational value. By challenging those with whom they work regarding 'their certitudes' (Freire 1997: 83), it is possible to extract educational outputs from almost any setting or experience. However, constantly demanding young people to justify their opinions and behaviour is a technique which has limited mileage. Therefore it is essential that workers construct opportunities for learning by initiating events, organising visits and distributing materials with the intention of stimulating conversation and directing the attention of young people towards the consideration of particular topics and subjects. Such interventions will by their very nature seek to encourage certain beliefs, attitudes and outcomes rather than others. As teachers and educators, rather than mere facilitators, youth workers engage in the process of selection, and in so doing aim to manage and control the learning of those young people with whom they work. The educational aims may be hidden behind a veil of activity and the voluntary involvement of the young people. Nevertheless, youth workers are exercising control as much as the traditional teacher. Moral education may not involve memorising rules and procedures but it does involve acquiring 'habits of conduct in the same way we acquire our native language' (Oakeshott 1962: 62): that is, by sharing experiences with people who behave in certain ways. Therefore, for exactly the same reasons that schoolteachers must justify the content of their lessons, so youth workers must be prepared to defend their interventions – to explain why they shape and manage the learning of others in particular ways.

Control in practice is part of youth workers' responsibility to ensure an appropriate learning environment is created. To this end workers and their managers or agencies make rules and plan programmes and activities (often in conjunction with young people). This is essentially about setting the scene for the work. During the course of the work occasions may also arise when workers may have to control or 'restrain' the young people with whom they work. There are at least four kinds of reasons workers may give for intervening to control the context of the work or the behaviour of particular young people, which we will describe briefly in turn: educational challenge; equality of access; equality of treatment; and the promotion of welfare.

1. Educational challenge

On the basis of their professional judgement, workers may intervene to maintain balance within the programme. Peters (1963) talks of the duty of the educator to 'initiate' young people into areas of knowledge they would not otherwise encounter. For example, a group of young people planning a series of activities may have exclusively chosen sports-related activities offered by a nearby leisure centre. If that occurs we might expect the worker to initiate a discussion about why they made these choices and offer alternatives such as a trip to a city farm, arts centre or dance studio to broaden the horizons of the young people.

2. Equality of access

Promotion of equality has often been viewed as one of the key aims of youth work practice. One of the ways in which this may be denied is if a particular project or centre works only with a small group of people, effectively excluding others who might benefit. Therefore a worker may intervene in a male-dominated centre which has a reputation for aggression and toughness in order to create an atmosphere more conducive to encouraging the participation of young women who are currently not members and are in effect being denied access to facilities.

3. Equality of treatment

Workers may intervene to prevent young people from victimising, bullying or harassing other individuals or groups. For example, a group of young Asian women participating in a project may face continuous racial jibes and taunts, which workers have a duty to challenge. The issue for the worker is when and how to challenge constructively and ensure those doing the taunting not only stop, but understand why it is wrong. Workers may sometimes have to exclude certain young people from a centre, event or meeting if their behaviour is unacceptable, because allowing them to stay, or giving them a lot of time and attention, would disadvantage others.

4. Promotion of welfare

Workers have a duty to their employers and parents to ensure the safety and well-being of participants in specific ways. They may also judge that they have a general duty to protect young people from harming themselves or others, particularly those who are vulnerable. This they may do, for example, through stopping a fight, or banning drugs and alcohol from premises. This kind of intervention may be straightforward in a case of obvious danger or infringement of a rule the worker believes in. In other cases there may be a fine line between respecting young people's freedom to make their own choices (including mistakes) and unwarranted interference and parentalism (see Banks 2004: 222; Banks 2009).

Practice for control

Control through education

Quite often reference is made to youth work as a form of social control, meaning that it is about socialising young people into modes of behaviour and responsible citizenship so that they fit into society. This is quite consistent with its educational purpose and in some ways, given our discussion above, it is difficult to dispute this claim. However, most youth workers would not identify this as the core purpose of their work, since there is a sense in which all those working in welfare occupations, including educators, are inevitably involved in transmitting prevailing values and norms, although some adopt a more critical approach than others. Youth workers would tend to stress the development of critical thinking, questioning, and extending young people's choices. They might talk more of participating in society than fitting in; about fostering democracy rather than responsibility (Jeffs 2001; Jeffs and Smith 2005). In so doing they would inevitably endeavour to transform the focus of debates about control from one which has largely been centred on how society might better manage and manipulate the behaviour of young people and others into one more concerned with how individuals as citizens rather than subjects might more forcefully engage with and challenge the state, those institutions they engage with, such as schools in the case of young people, and their social environment.

It is important for workers to be aware that neither the work they are doing nor the role of an educator is neutral; that education can be a force for challenge and change or for fortifying the status quo. Most workers are clear that youth work is not about indoctrination or brainwashing. Arguably these would not be defined as education in the strict sense. Although there is no doubt that what passes for or has passed itself off as 'education' has frequently had such goals in mind. The potential for the misuse of the role of educator is great – as Green (Chapter 8) discusses in relation to religious conversion. Increasingly, though, the danger within both the formal and informal sectors appears to emanate not from rogue educators seeking to indoctrinate young people and convert them to a particular religious or political viewpoint, but from a highly centralised state determined to restrict the educational experience to what it deems useful, worthwhile and safe. Within the formal sector the British government moved relentlessly from imposing a National Curriculum, without even a token consultation with teachers, to the production of national textbooks in English, maths, design and technology, science, history and geography. This approach, by denying the teacher and the student the opportunity to assemble a curriculum, or even to negotiate sequence, effectively reduces the role of the former to that of an instructor. It closes down dialogue and restricts negotiation to fringe issues, as control over what is to be taught (the curriculum) is transferred to distant experts, politicians and funders.

Youth workers still retain marginally greater freedom from bureaucratic control than their colleagues in the school sector. The nature of the contact certainly means they have more space and time for conversation and dialogue and greater opportunities to allow young people the opportunity to shape the conversation (Hirsch 2005). However, the growth of commissioning and targetted funding increasingly means that youth workers must 'deliver' training and pre-packaged materials designed to reduce teenage pregnancy, antisocial behaviour, obesity or whatever the latest moral panic deems important. Whole swathes of the statutory and voluntary sectors are now funding-led in ways that have eroded the historical autonomy that allowed the educational content of youth work to be shaped by dialogue and in part determined via negotiation. It has been replaced with a practice that is as narrow and qualification-driven as the diet young people are force-fed in schools and colleges. Funders are seeking to impose conditions that require workers to show they have reduced offending, antisocial behaviour or risk activities in a given area. Pre-packaged programmes or 'curriculum units' are also increasingly being provided by some employers who make their use mandatory. Such changes, such as those forced upon schoolteachers, may be opposed by educators and young people alike but the pressures to conform in the name of efficiency and effectiveness are immense. Punitive financial penalties in particular impose either conformity or a requirement that workers lie about outcomes and the work undertaken to secure a continuation of funding. This fosters an approach to the work where 'getting through the programme becomes the end' and to which the understanding of the young person becomes 'subordinated' (Haynes 1998: 49).

Pockets of what may be termed 'traditional practice' remain that enable young people to become partners within the enterprise rather than clients or customers, and settings that give workers the ability to choose both what and how they wish to teach. An autonomy that allows them, if they so wish, to create what Haynes terms a 'community of enquiry' (1998: 133) – space where young people can construct programmes and create experiences of shared communal learning, which can respond directly to the expressed needs of the participants. Overwhelmingly such youth work takes place in small voluntary and faith-based units or on the street where it is more difficult for managers to monitor the practice of workers. Workers in such settings are better equipped to resist the growing pressure to formalise youth work, create chains of command and produce identifiable outcomes that have eroded the capacity of workers to structure communities of enquiry. However, top-down clamouring for registration of all British youth workers and centres threatens even this limited sovereignty (Clubs for Young People 2009).

Control by diversion and prevention

The third sense of youth work as control has a more direct relationship to the maintenance of public order – the prevention and diversion of young people from trouble, crime and causing disturbance. This version of youth work as control would regard the achievement of such outcomes either as the core purpose, or one of the main purposes of youth work. Using youth work methods – informal educational processes – the aim is to reduce or prevent truancy, offending, teenage pregnancies, or any other of the myriad social problems thought to be caused by 'out-of-control' young people. Recently there has been a growth of youth work in these fields, with many specialised projects being established which stress this approach either in their titles or in their stated aims of 'diversion from crime', 'alternatives to custody' or 'truancy reduction'. Much of this work is designed to remove young people from the streets. In the most extreme forms youth workers are being asked to help enforce curfews and assist in 'truancy sweeps' (DfES 2002; Home Office 2001). Both activities raise ethical issues regarding the basis on which young people, purely in terms of their age, are being denied freedom of movement. Predictably this has led to a muted debate as to whether youth work agencies should participate in such projects (Waiton 2007a, 2007b).

Youth crime prevention work is a particularly interesting example, with some commentators suggesting that the youth service should 'welcome opportunities to become involved more explicitly in preventing youth crime, that there is encouraging evidence that it can do so successfully' (Smith and Paylor 1997: 17) and that youth workers 'should see this as a "window of opportunity" to create a clear role for themselves in future initiatives' (France and Wiles 1997: 13). On the other hand, Jeffs and Smith (2008, 1994: 25) warn against the gradual replacement of the educational orientation of most youth work initiatives by control, identifying a drift towards a 'new authoritarianism' forcing workers increasingly into 'modes of intervention located within a tradition of behaviour modification rather than education for autonomy and choice'.

Both of these positions seem somewhat extreme. There certainly is a danger of the new authoritarianism pushing youth work towards the control end of the spectrum. Funding and work are increasingly targeted on those perceived to be most 'at risk' or problematic (see Chapters 2 and 4). Yet it is interesting that youth work funded specifically with a crime prevention remit does not generally use behaviour modification techniques, manipulation or authoritarian rules. Youth workers recognise that they are not the police, probation officers or social workers. They know that if they embrace the crime control agenda too overtly and directly, then there is a danger that they cease to be youth workers; that they will be tempted, or pushed, to use a range of methods and techniques not usually associated with youth work to achieve the outcomes required by their sponsors or employers. By doing that, they are in danger of not only losing whatever precarious identity they hold as youth workers, but risk failing in the task set by their funders or sponsors. For the reason why youth work may be successful in working with young people categorised as 'at risk' is precisely because it does so in an informal and participative way; that it tends to work alongside and with young people and listen to their concerns and needs. As soon as the workers become overly preoccupied with achieving prescribed outputs and monitoring and evaluating their results, their primary focus is distracted from the young people, and their work can become less effective. This is not to say that workers should not evaluate the impact of their work, but it may explain some of their reluctance to do so. Contemporary funding mechanisms and the 'audit culture' lay great emphasis upon the measurement of outcomes and external evaluation. The data flow in relation to 'achieved outcomes', but what is interesting is that youth workers' own accounts of their work speak instead of building relationships based on mutual trust, faciliting the learning of young people, and engaging in challenging and confidence-building activities (Spence *et al.* 2007).

A demarcation line, however ill-defined at times, does exist between those employed to control the criminal activities of young people, such as crime prevention officers or security officers patrolling a shopping precinct, and a detached youth worker. All three may operate in the same locality, focus their attention on young people, seek out their company and engage in conversation with them. However, their reasons for doing so vary enormously. For the first two the purpose is to prevent the young people from committing crime. Therefore they have no professional interest in those who 'behave' except as potential deviants or purveyors of information about criminal peers. Youth workers operate according to different criteria. For them any decision to focus attention on one segment of the youth population in the area must be justified according to need. They must be able to give reasons for targeting on the basis of professional judgement that takes full account of who will benefit most from their intervention and where the greatest need resides.

The second reason why targeting those misbehaving jeopardises the distinctiveness of youth work relates to the educational process itself. Although youth workers may run programmes and initiate activities, these are not their prime purpose. They are the means whereby opportunities for dialogue and conversation can be engendered, through which the worker can express concern for young people, indicate interest in them as people, display trust and respect, and show that they value them as individuals. However, such relationships must be open and honest. Dialogue, as opposed to instruction, requires the worker to treat young people as worthy of respect. Respect may be regarded as an 'active sympathy' towards another human being (Downie and Telfer 1969, 1980). In the Kantian sense, this human being is a person who has desires and hopes and is capable of making choices, and therefore should never be treated simply as a means to our ends (Kant 1964: 32–33). Whatever the differences in age, income or background, the worker has to be with that person, rather than seeking merely to act upon them. This is crucial. If the worker enters into dialogue with the desire merely to act upon those with whom they are working, they are perceiving them as an object rather than as a person. When this is the case then the relationship is wholly or partially closed to interaction (Jeffs and Smith 2005).

In the absence of mutual respect, genuine dialogue – when individuals share ideas and are simultaneously open to the views of others – ceases to be tenable. For mutual respect cannot long survive within relationships where one party holds themselves morally, intellectually and ethically superior to the other. Within such a climate informal educators would be unable to justify a *modus operandi* based on a belief that they are engaging with equals. Their faith in the potential of education via dialogue and conversation would consequently be shown to have been profoundly misplaced. They would be left with no choice but to opt for more formal and structured modes of intervention – programmes of instruction based on the sort of implicit contract which club and centre workers often strike, where they offer 'clients' access to leisure facilities or welfare services in return for participation in morally improving programmes. This type of approach is one where the ends (better behaviour) would be used to justify the means (formal contracts).

The application of youth work techniques to crime prevention work is not something which most workers would find intrinsically unacceptable. Indeed, as an alternative to military-style policing operations, the arbitrary exclusion of young people from public space and the use of gratuitous violence against potential offenders to discourage their presence, it would be an attractive option.

Furthermore, if their introduction precipitates a decline in offending behaviour then this is something again which most would surely welcome. However, the question remains whether the adoption of specific techniques and styles of practice (informal educational methods) can transform crime management or prevention programmes into youth work. If the core purpose of the work ceases to be education, and the values relating to respect, equality of opportunity and participation are lost, then it is doubtful.

Yet there is no doubt that at a micro-level of day-to-day practice most workers on such projects are still doing what we would recognise as youth work and are relating to young people as educators (Crimmens *et al.* 2004; Spence *et al.* 2007). However, at a macro-level, the policy and funding framework within which they are doing this has a utilitarian stress upon outcomes relating to the control and management of dangerous and threatening youth. State welfare workers have always had to manage the tension between developing autonomy and control; and as long as autonomy at the micro-level showed up as control at the macro-level, everybody was satisfied. However, workers are now being asked to prove this link. This threatens the educational purpose and approach of their work. They are being asked to make explicit what was hitherto accepted as implicit. They are being asked to state as a core purpose what was once regarded as a desirable by-product. The policy and funding framework is no longer a rather distant set of limits which can be left to managers, but is something that has become intertwined with the everyday work. What was once experienced as a cocoon seems now to be more like a spider's web. Before they become hopelessly enmeshed, youth workers and youth work managers need to stop and take serious stock of where the silken trail is leading them.

The question as to whether the youth service and youth workers should eschew work focusing specifically upon changing the behaviour of 'problematic' groups and keep their hands 'clean' is not a simple one to answer. It will depend upon the outcomes expected of the work and the extent to which workers may have to target their work and use alien techniques. Mounting governmental concern relating to an assumed rise in levels of youth offending and the appearance of what has been dubbed an 'underclass' has led to a marked shift in the allocation of funding to projects which claim to manage and control 'disaffected youth' (DCSF 2008; Jeffs 1997a, 1997b; Jeffs and Smith 1994). As is noted by Jeffs and Smith in Chapter 4 on funding, the growing use of targeted funding poses a dilemma for youth workers. It is creating new jobs for them and providing resources. However, in return it requires youth workers to set aside their professional judgement regarding with whom they ought to work. Where the focus is upon control then inevitably those who pose the least threat will receive the least attention. This will mean the neglect of work with those who tend to be less visible, less troublesome and less demanding. Where does this leave work with young women (except as potential teenage mothers or drug users), with lesbian, gay or bisexual young people (except as potential victims of AIDS) or with young people with disabilities, for example? These are serious ethical issues for workers as well as for policy-makers and funders. It is important that youth workers challenge policies and practices that are regarded as discriminatory or harmful to young people. Indeed, The NYA statement on ethical conduct in youth work includes the promotion of social justice for young people and in society more generally as one of the four key ethical principles in youth work, which includes 'drawing attention to unjust policies and practices and actively seeking to change them' (NYA 2004: par. 5.1.4).

Conclusion

The issue of control in youth work always has been and will continue to be the source of many ethical debates and practice dilemmas. What we have called 'control in practice' is essential for all good educational work – involving workers in careful planning of the learning process as they tread a line between the extremes of authoritarian and permissive methods of working – balancing the controlling curriculum with the casual conversation. It is an issue that needs much further exploration and discussion, since it is at the heart of youth work practice.

On the other hand, the lengthy arguments of academics about the dangers of practice for control may seem irrelevant, or a luxury, to practitioners working with young people on the streets, searching for the next source of funding or fighting against the closure of a project. We are not suggesting that workers deny the impact of their work upon crime reduction, drug abuse or unemployment. Control and management of dangerous and threatening youth has always underpinned much youth work. First, this is because funders frequently require it to do so. Welfare agencies such as health authorities, housing associations or children's services expect their investment to produce a reduction in the future demand for their services and changes in behaviour, while local councillors and community groups generally expect to see the efforts of youth workers translated into lower rates of offending and fewer 'kids on the streets' and 'hanging around'. Second, the public also often expect it to address problems such as 'delinquency' and 'young people making a nuisance of themselves'.

Workers can feel vulnerable to such demands because they are aware that the public and other welfare workers habitually misunderstand their role, perceiving them as leisure workers who in the words of one teacher are running 'about playing with bairns all day, and getting paid for it' (Moir 1997: 5). Inevitably workers may fall into line pleading for funds and support on the grounds that they reduce offending and raise the behaviourial norms of young people.

Implicit within the activity of youth work is a normative belief that it will confer benefits upon those who come into contact with the worker; that it will make them better rather than worse people; and more educated and more socially responsible rather than less. It is assumed that youth work will help make them better citizens – individuals who would be more likely to respect the law and behave in morally acceptable ways. All worthwhile education must in the final analysis be an act of faith. The alternative is to teach only what can be measured and enumerated.

If youth work is, as we believe, an educational activity, we must learn to trust practitioners and participants mutually to create worthwhile experiences. Funders, managers and the rest of us must resist the temptation to impose a control agenda upon them. We must allow youth workers the freedom to initiate young people into modes of thought, activities and disciplines they would otherwise be denied or would find it difficult to assimilate or engage in unaided. We must allow them to act according to the principles and modes of conduct that are incumbent on youth workers as a consequence of them becoming youth workers as opposed to being, for example, school-teachers, street wardens or police officers. Decisions, ethical or otherwise, regarding what are and are not worthwhile modes of thought and activities must be left to practitioners, although they are clearly obligated to engage in dialogue with young people, parents, funders and the wider community if they are to make informed choices. Youth work, as Peters (1959: 97) explains, is essentially a process that seeks to introduce people 'to what is valuable in an intelligible and voluntary manner'. It is the educational purpose that delineates youth work from the mere provision of leisure activities, and also draws a sharp line between youth work and those interventions designed primarily to entertain, control, manage and contain young people. Consequently work with young people that sets out specifically to tackle offending and delinquency, to keep young people off the streets or to allow their parents or guardians to leave them somewhere 'safe' with the aim of controlling and containing rather than educating, swiftly ceases to be youth work.

Questions for reflection and discussion

1   Do you find the distinction between 'practice for control' and 'control in practice' a useful one? Can you give examples from your own experience?

2   Do you think the presence of surveillance cameras in settings where youth work takes place constrains open and honest dialogue between youth workers and young people, or do cameras contribute to creating safe spaces for young people and adults?

3   Youth workers are increasingly being required to target those young people who are regarded as 'misbehaving' or as at risk of behaving in ways that are regarded as harmful to themselves or to others. Do you think this is a legitimate role for youth workers? What does this mean for the traditional concept of youth work as a universal service, based upon voluntary relationships with young people?

Recommended reading

Davies, B. (2008) *The New Labour Years: A History of the Youth Service in England 1997–2007*, Leicester: The National Youth Agency. This is the third volume of Davies's history of the youth service, which covers a key period when a focus on targeting, outcomes, measurement and control of young people gained momentum in England.

Youth and Policy (2008), Issue 100 (published by The National Youth Agency). The hundredth anniversary issue of the journal, *Youth and Policy*, contains a number of useful articles reflecting on the current state of youth work.

References

Baden-Powell, R. (1908) *Scouting For Boys*, London: Arthur Pearson.

Banks, S. (2004) 'The dilemmas of intervention', in J. Roche and S. Tucker (eds) *Youth in Society*, 2nd edn, London: Sage/Open University Press.

Banks, S. (2009) 'Values and ethics in work with young people', in J. Wood and J. Hine (eds) *Work with Young People: Developments in Theory, Policy and Practice*, London: Sage.

Bickerdike, K.C. (1926) *The Church and the Boy Outside*, London: Wells Gardner, Darton & Co.

Clubs for Young People (2009) *A Blueprint for 21st Century Youth Clubs*, London: Clubs for Young People.

Collingwood, J. and Collingwood, M. (1990) *Hannah More*, Oxford: Lion Publishing.

Corrigan, P. and Leonard, P. (1978) *Social Work Practice under Capitalism: A Marxist Approach*, London: Macmillan.

Crimmens, D., Factor, F., Jeffs, T., Pitts, J., Pugh, C., Spence, J. and Turner, P. (2004) *Reaching Socially Excluded Young People: A National Study of Street-based Youth Work*, York: Joseph Rowntree Foundation.

Davies, B. (2008) *The New Labour Years: A History of the Youth Service in England 1997–2007*, Leicester: The National Youth Agency.

Davies, B. (2009) 'Squaring the circle? The state of youth work in some children and young people's services' *Youth and Policy*, 103: 5–24.

Davin, A. (1996) *Growing Up Poor: Home, School and Street in London 1870–1914*, London: Rivers of Oram Press.

Department for Education and Skills (DfES) (2002) *Guidlines for Truancy Sweeps*, London: DfES.

Department for Children, Schools and Families (DCSF) (2008) *Targeted Youth Support: Intregrated Support for Vulnerable Young People*, London: DCSF.

de St Croix, T. (2008) 'Informal educators or bureaucrats and spies?', *Youth Work Now*, December: 12.

de St Croix, T. (2009) ' "Forgotten corners": a reflection on radical youth work in Britain, 1940–1990', in R. Gilchrist, T. Jeffs, J. Spence and J. Walker (eds) *Essays in the History of Youth and Community Work: Discovering the Past*, Lyme Regis: Russell House.

Downie, R. and Telfer, E. (1969) *Respect for Persons*, London: Routledge & Kegan Paul.

—— (1980) *Caring and Curing*, London: Methuen.

Ford, K., Hunter, R., Merton, B. and Waller, D. (2002) *Transforming Youth Work Management Programme Course Reader*, London: fpm.

France, A. and Wiles, P. (1996) *The Youth Action Scheme – A Report of the National Evaluation*, London: Department for Education and Employment.

—— (1997) 'The Youth Action Scheme and the future of youth work', *Youth and Policy*, 57: 1–16.

Freire, P. (1997) *Pedagogy of Hope. Reliving Pedagogy of the Oppressed*, New York: Continuum.

Furedi, F. (1997) *Culture of Fear: Risk-taking and the Morality of Low Expectations*, London: Cassell.

Gate, E.M. (1933) *Roland Philipps: Boy Scout*, London: Roland House.

Haynes, F. (1998) *The Ethical School*, London: Routledge.

Hirsch, B. (2005) *A Place to Call Home: After-school Programs for Urban Youth*, New York: Teachers College Press.

Home Office (2001) *Checklist for Police and Schools Working Together to Tackle Truancy, Crime and Disorder*, London: Home Office.

Hurt, J.S. (1979) *Elementary Schooling and the Working Classes 1860–1918*, London: Routledge & Kegan Paul.

Jeffs, T. (1997a) 'Changing their ways: youth work and the "underclass theory"', in R. MacDonald (ed.) *Youth, the Underclass and Social Exclusion*, London: Routledge.

—— (1997b) 'Wild things? Young people our new enemy within', *Concept*, 8: 4–8.

—— (2001) 'Citizenship, youth work and democratic renewal', *Scottish Youth Issues Journal*, 3: 11–34.

—— (2004) 'Curriculum debate: a letter to Jon Ord', *Youth and Policy*, 84: 55–62.

Jeffs, T. and Smith, M.K. (1994) 'Young people, youth work and a new authoritarianism', *Youth and Policy*, 46: 17–32.

—— (1996) '"Getting the dirtbags off the streets". Curfews and other solutions to juvenile crime', *Youth and Policy*, 53: 1–14.

—— (2005) *Informal Education*, 3rd edn, Ticknall, Derbyshire: Education Now Books.

—— (2008) 'Valuing youth work', *Youth and Policy*, 100: 277–302.

Jephcott, P. (1942) *Girls Growing Up*, London: Faber and Faber.

Jolly, J. (2009) 'Is the concept of youth work hard to grasp?', *Youth Work Now*, 9 August.

Kant, I. (1964) *Groundwork of the Metaphysics of Morals*, New York: Harper & Row.

Kingman, J.M. and Sidman, E. (1935) *A Manual of Settlement Boys' Work*, Boston, MA: National Federation of Settlements.

Langan, M. and Lee, P. (eds) (1989) *Radical Social Work Today*, London: Unwin Hyman.

Lewin, K., Lippitt, R. and White, R. (1939) 'Patterns of aggressive behaviour in experimentally created social climates', *Journal of Social Psychology*, 10: 347–357.

Moir, S. (1997) 'Theory and practice: towards a critical pedagogy of youth work', *Concept*, 7: 5–7.

National Youth Agency (NYA) (2004) *Ethical Conduct in Youth Work: A Statement of Values and Principles from the National Youth Agency*, Leicester: National Youth Agency.

Oakeshott, M. (1962) *Rationalism in Politics*, New York: Basic Books.

Ord, J. (2009) 'Thinking the unthinkable: youth work without voluntary participation?' *Youth and Policy*, 103: 39–48, 103.

Peters, R.S. (1959) *Authority, Responsibility and Education*, London: Unwin.

Peters, R.S. (1963) *Education as Initiation*, London: Evans Brothers.

Rawls, J. (1951) 'Outline for a decision procedure for ethics', *Philosophical Review*, 60: 177–197.

Rawls, J. (1999) *A Theory of Justice* (revised edn), Cambridge, MA: Harvard University Press.

Robertson, S. (2005) *Youth Clubs: Association, Participation, Friendship and Fun*, Lyme Regis: Russell House.

Russell, B. (1932) *Education and the Social Order*, London: Unwin.

Russell, C. and Russell, L. (1932) *Lads' Clubs: Their History, Organisation and Management*, London: A.C. Black.

Sapin, K. (2009) *Essential Skills for Youth Work Practice*, London: Sage.

Secretan, R. (1931) *London Below Bridges*, London: Godfrey Bles.

Shepherd, J. (2009) 'Someone to watch over you', *Education Guardian,* 4 August: 1–2.

Shotton, J. (1993) *No Master High or Low: Libertarian Education and Schooling 1890–1990*, Bristol: Libertarian Education.

Smith, M. (1994) *Local Education. Community, Conversation, Praxis*, Buckingham: Open University Press.

Smith, D. and Paylor, I. (1997) 'Reluctant heroes: youth workers and crime prevention', *Youth and Policy*, 57: 17–28.

Spence, J. and Devanney, C. with Noonan, K. (2007) *Youth Work: Voices of Practice*, Leicester: The National Youth Agency.

Waiton, S. (2007a) *Scared of the Kids: Curfews, Crime and the Regulation of Young People*, Dundee: University of Abertay Dundee Press.

Waiton, S. (2007b) *The Politics of Antisocial Behaviour: Amoral Panics*, London: Routledge.

8

Youth workers as converters?

Ethical issues in faith-based youth work

Maxine Green

Introduction

In the past 20 years there has been a rise in the number of youth workers being employed by faith organisations in Britain. This has been accompanied by institutions offering faith-based training and providing forums to debate the ethical considerations accompanying this training. The literature also reflects these trends, with expositions on interfaith work, spiritual development and how this affects the political context. The range of faith-based employment for youth workers has also expanded from 'a youth worker for our place of worship' to a whole host of project work where issues of faith are central to the role of youth workers. It is where youth work meets faith that ethical issues emerge that have to be discussed. 'Youth workers as converters' is a very powerful concept. It invokes a whole range of assumptions about the role of youth workers and the outcomes of the youth work they undertake. As more and more youth workers are appointed in faith-based settings this is no longer of marginal interest but affects a considerable proportion of all professional youth workers employed.

Debates about the nature and value of faith-based youth work often cover strongly held beliefs which need to be explored and challenged: for example, the concept of conversion can be regarded negatively as an act of coercion, or positively as fulfilling human potential. It is rare to have a genuine dialogue which encompasses the possibility of both being true in different circumstances, and what often happens in discussing faith and religion is that the arguments polarise into good versus bad or right versus wrong. Constructive dialogue in matters of faith occurs most effectively when people feel safe enough to leave the moral high ground and seek the interesting middle ground where particular issues can be explored and discussed.

The approach of this chapter is to name the polarities, identify the middle ground and explore the ethical issues as they are worked out there. It aims to explore some of the background against which these assumptions are made. It will explore the ethical issues, both for faith-based youth work and for the professional youth worker. The chapter demonstrates that ideologically inspired youth work raises complex questions and careful thought is needed to avoid the 'knee-jerk' reaction that often accompanies this debate. The intention is not to devise a code of practice for faith-based or political youth work, but to raise the ethical issues that surround such work. To develop good practice in work that is both faith based and secular it is important that a rigorous and challenging dialogue is encouraged.

Conversion

'Conversion' is a form of change and it is undeniable that change is expected in youth work. The question is: what sort of change and conversion is appropriate and what is the role of the youth worker as a professional in that change? Conversion in the religious sense can be a climactic, charismatic experience where people feel a deep calling to which they respond positively; it can also be a slower, more cumulative process where a belief is gathered until the person can declare their faith. In either case the youth worker can accompany young people and support the transition and the choices they make. Young people sometimes 'find' a vocational call which transports them, for example if they fall in love or want to join the army, where the youth worker may not share the aspiration for the young person but accompanies them through the process. What is important is that the concept of conversion is not necessarily positive or negative. It is possible to assess the impact that conversion has on people's lives and to make judgements based on assessing their subsequent behaviour against particular expectations. For example, as a result of conversion, are people happier, and do they have more or less control over their lives?

It is also important to widen the concept of conversion so that it embraces other meaningful life changes. The current climate in education is risk averse and much happier with slow, incremental change. Youth work has a practice of taking young people out of their comfort zones, especially using the outdoors. By giving them a huge change in their experience, youth work can enable them to make large shifts in their learning and knowledge of themselves. Conversion in a faith sense offers a similar paradigm shift in experience and should not be avoided because of its potentially spectacular effect.

What is faith-based youth work?

There is no one model of faith-based youth work. Different major faiths and denominations use different methods to achieve different aims, and this work has varied over time and ranges from best practice to very poor practice. There is no doubt that at the 'poor practice' end of the spectrum there has been considerable abuse of young people, where powerful concepts of salvation and the after-life have been used to instil regimented, unthinking following. In social science, Freud (1927) saw religion as a means of controlling the masses who were unable to internalise the concept of self-realisation, and Marx (1938) saw it as 'the opium of the people' which mystified citizens into accepting subjugation. Work with people that draws upon ideological and religious frameworks is exceptionally powerful and as such is open to abuse as well as use.

This concern is particularly important in the context of fears about the radicalisation of young people by fundamentalist faith sectors. Although much teaching in fundamentalism is didactic and cannot be seen as youth work, a youth worker within this set-up may be seen as a role model and can build relationships and trust with young people. The art of reflective practice together with familiarity with the broad empowering values of youth work have the potential of adding critical dialogue into extreme situations and bringing reason and choice to the young person.

In a more positive frame, people of faith have inspired and campaigned for huge changes in social reform, welfare and education; for example, Jewish and Christian organisations were at the forefront of the foundation of the youth service in Britain and subsequent developments, as these quotations illustrate:

> The 'youth service' in England developed in the late nineteenth century. The earliest voluntary youth organisations were started by philanthropic individuals, many of whom were Christian. The Young Men's Christian Association (YMCA) and the Girls' Friendly Society are amongst those that aimed to provide education and leisure opportunities for young workers. In the second half of the century charity work on behalf of working young people mushroomed and was led by city centre evangelical missions and ragged schools where clubs for young people began to be formed. In 1884 there were 300 institutes and working boys clubs in the Diocese of London alone and most of these were associated with churches.
>
> (Church of England 1996: 148)

> It is important to note that the Church of England, at local, regional and national level, has played a significant role in supporting, contributing to and, in many instances pioneering a wide range of youth work initiatives. Notable among these pioneering aspects which influenced subsequent statutory provision have been the numerous city centre-based detached youth projects; night shelters for the young; hostel accommodation schemes for unmarried young mothers; motor car and bike projects and innovative schemes of training for part-time youth workers.
>
> (Church of England 1996: 150)

The first Jewish youth club established in Britain was the German Street Girls Club in London's East End in 1883, and had as its aspiration the integration of young, newly immigrated, Eastern European Jews into mainstream British Society.

(Rose 2005: 3)

This influence continues in the present both through existing structures and with the rapid increase in the number of faith organisations that are employing full-time and part-time youth workers.

Specialist professional qualifying programmes have been established in Christian and Muslim youth work and there is a growth of interest in the role of youth work in many other faiths (Ahmed *et al.* 2007); while the Jewish faith has had a long history of training for faith-based youth work. There are several reasons behind this shift to employing more faith-based youth workers. These include the institutions being concerned about the reduced number of young people joining as full members and wanting to ensure that faith is passed on to the younger generation. There is an awareness of the 'spiritual rights' of young people and a desire to empower them by giving them access to their spiritual heritage. This investment in the future also extends to wanting the best for society and ensuring that the faith perspective is not lost. There is also a desire for the institution to continue and an understanding that this demands new members. Many religious institutions have focused on young people, since they recognise adolescence as being a critical period for faith development and they plan their work programme to reflect this. The concern to prevent and combat radicalisation and extremism has also encouraged agencies to employ youth workers to bring a moderating influence. This is especially apparent in the Muslim context (Hamid 2006) and is discussed more fully in Chapter 9.

Educating the 'next generation' is part of the responsibility of a society and it is essential that skills, knowledge and values be passed on to young people to equip the community as a whole. It is particularly important for religious movements to be able to offer their history and practice to young people. Failure to pass on these ideas not only injures the organisations, but also disempowers young people who are then unable to build on previous work. Western societies accept the responsibility to 'educate' young people by providing opportunities for them to become literate, numerate and to gain an understanding of the world. There is commitment by some societies to spiritual development as part of the whole education agenda. In Britain youth work reports have included reference to spirituality since 1944; for example, in 1969 Lord Redcliffe-Maud defined the aim of youth services as:

To offer individual young people in their leisure time, opportunities to discover and develop their personal resources of body, mind and spirit and thus equip themselves to live the life of mature, creative and responsible members of a free society.

(HMSO 1969: 55)

The rights of young people for religious education accompany the responsibility of organisations to offer their thinking and practice to the 'next generation'. This does not mean that young people should be 'trained', inducted or programmed, but that they have a chance to become familiar with different life frameworks. The preciousness of these life frameworks is not generally accepted in the 'over-developed' world, in contrast to some older societies, for example, the Seneca of North America (Wallace 1972), where receiving knowledge of myth and ritual is seen as a privilege.

The report *How Faith Grows* (Church of England 1991) describes different theories of faith development and 'stages' which people pass through as they acquire a faith. 'Stage three' details a wish to belong to a faith crowd or current, where many people join together in sharing belief and practice. This stage occurs commonly at the time of adolescence when existentialist questions are asked along with a search for a future adult identity. Young people are particularly vulnerable at this time to groups who give them a sense of belonging and being loved. In the worst cases this need is exploited unscrupulously with fundamentalists of many faiths targeting young people. There has been a resistance to this from youth workers in the Muslim community who have aimed to set up alternative provision and support to counter extremists who have targeted young Muslim men (Hamid 2006).

Young people have a right to the theological and political tools to enable them to make choices about different groups. Experiences of responsible organisations can give them balanced life frameworks by which they can assess new groups they may encounter so that they may approach these groups with reason and caution. It is important where there is a will to pass on skills, beliefs and experience that this is done in a way that empowers young people. There is a real difference between good youth work that gives young people increased opportunities, and indoctrination and coercion (Green 1997). It is especially important for religious organisations that have centuries of experience of 'conversion' not to abuse this knowledge, as they offer opportunities of spiritual and political development to young people. This is even more pertinent where falling numbers may endanger the life of the institution itself and the need for members becomes a primary aim.

The ethics of youth work in faith-based organisations

The youth worker is often the catalyst between the traditional society and young people. By working alongside young people the youth worker can enable political, social or religious debate, and thus offer a forum in which this development can take place. This is an essential role, both for the society and the rights of young people.

The ethical issues that surround youth work relate to how this process occurs. Clarity is needed about what sort of ideological youth work constitutes good practice and whether there is some work undertaken with young people that is unethical. The first issue is to establish what is 'good youth work'. Banks (1996, 2009) has supported increased opportunities to debate professional values and practice and cites how institutions such as the English National Youth Agency (NYA) and the Community and Youth Workers' Union have drawn up guidelines and codes of ethics or conduct. The National Youth Agency in England (2004) statement on ethical conduct includes four ethical and five professional principles. Banks (2009) has summarised the five professional principles under one heading entitled 'Act with professional integrity', and outlines the NYA principles as follows:

1 Treat young people with respect, valuing each individual and avoiding negative discrimination.
2 Respect and promote young people's rights to make their own decisions and choices, unless the welfare or legitimate interests of themselves or others is seriously threatened.
3 Promote and ensure the welfare and safety of young people while permitting them to learn through undertaking challenging educational activities.
4 Contribute towards the promotion of social justice for young people and in society generally, through encouraging respect for difference and diversity and challenging discrimination.
5 Act with professional integrity.

I will use these principles as a basis of good youth work practice to reflect on a hypothetical scene within a Christian youth work project and from this draw out particular ethical issues in faith-based youth work.

Case study 8.1

The situation involves a young woman, Sheri, coming to a youth worker, Jim, wanting help. She explains that she is depressed; she is having problems with a relationship and with her parents.

1 If an informal education model is used Jim will help Sheri explore and analyse the situation. This will be by using open questions that will enable Sheri to think of all the aspects relating to her circumstances.

Jim will encourage this divergent exploration and the ownership of the problem will remain with Sheri. Afterwards, Jim will help Sheri sum up the range of options open to her and explore the 'pros and cons' of each option. Sheri can then reject the least suitable options and decide on a course of action. Jim can then help Sheri identify the resources she needs to enable that change. Sheri can then go and do what she has decided. Another way that Jim can be helpful to her is by being there to debrief the course of action and to enable Sheri to analyse the situation for future development.

2 A more directive approach may occur when a worker has a strong single framework that he uses in all situations. In this case when Sheri approaches Jim he is already making decisions about Sheri in relation to his own framework, considering, for example: 'Is she a Christian?' 'Is she saved?' Jim will then hear the situation within this framework. Although the worker may listen carefully to Sheri, there may be a script at the back of his mind which impairs the informal education process. Thus Sheri's 'problem' may be seen in terms of Jim's faith and he will use his understanding of his faith to solve the problem rather than enable Sheri to address the problem as she sees it. The process is much more likely to be like a consultation where Sheri lays out the situation, Jim ponders and comes up with a solution that is 'sold' to Sheri, and then takes some responsibility in enabling this solution to happen. Jim may continue to work to reinforce and support Sheri, encouraging her to adopt his own ideological or religious framework.

3 A still more limiting approach is where a single solution is seen as the answer to all Sheri's problems. Here Jim may be so set on fulfilling his own agenda to 'bring Sheri to faith' that he is unable to hear her particular issues and will entreat Sheri to 'take Jesus as her personal saviour' and convince her that all will be well after making such a decision.

In the first scenario Jim is working within the NYA principles. Jim treats Sheri with respect and is helping her to make her own decisions and choices. The power is left with Sheri and the youth worker, Jim, takes the facilitating role. A good youth worker will be able to help the young person come up with a divergent range of possible outcomes which may meet the young person's enquiry or need. Although the youth worker will have his or her own values and experience, the most important aspect of this work is that the young person is given space to explore options, is supported while she makes choices and is empowered to develop through the experience.

In the second scenario the worker's own values have framed the encounter. The worker has allowed his own values to frame the problem and decrease the range of options that Sheri has available to her. The exploratory nature of the process is impaired and the worker disempowers Sheri by taking her problem away and 'solving it', and thus not allowing Sheri to develop and grow from the experience. This is directly contrary to the second principle in the NYA statement that the youth worker should respect and promote young people's rights to make their own decisions. It also impacts upon the first principle where it seems that Sheri's own sense of value is being overpowered by Jim's understanding of what is right thinking.

In the third scenario the needs of the worker to convert Sheri are so strong that the whole informal education process is bypassed, and instead of enabling Sheri to address the problems that she faces, the agenda becomes that of the worker, Jim. Sheri is not empowered and is not able to use her situation to develop. Jim is not respecting or valuing Sheri here, and is not helping her in making her own decision. Insofar as Jim is exploiting the relationship and not recognising boundaries between personal and professional life, he is also failing to act with professional integrity.

Where there is an aim to convert or evangelise there is tremendous pressure not to take the 'risk' of exploring a divergent range of choices with the young person but to present a single viewpoint or solution. This is even stronger when the faith of the youth workers is very powerful in their own lives and may have led them to a vivid and personal transformation, which they want to share. This may mean that the work is based on a behavioural model with the young people being rewarded for making certain choices and electing to adopt the values of the institution. These rewards can be linked to a sense of belonging and worth which is a strong motivator for young people as they move towards an adult identity. Although the short-term effects of this sort of work can be dramatic it is questionable what sort of attitude change there is in the long term. Many dynamic evangelistic events, for example, using multi-media concert techniques, produce dramatic conversions that may be short-lived compared to a more reasoned faith acquired through a more open informal education process. There is a question concerning the efficacy of behavioural models of conversion. However, it is still the case that whatever the motives, youth work must be participative and empowering. 'Solving the problem' for a young person by offering a single religious or political solution or the conditional offer of belonging in exchange for membership is not informal education and is not youth work.

Everyone has a belief system

Although a committed or visionary youth worker has a more overt belief system, no youth workers are ideologically blank and devoid of personal values, and these will undoubtedly inform their work. A common position is to view youth work as having an ideologically neutral value base and to see a faith value base as being at best additional to this and at worst contrary to youth work values. Given this standpoint it then falls upon faith-based workers to defend their value base. However, this is a weak position and I contend that all youth workers should consider how their personal values impinge upon the work and what is professionally valid. A notable addition to faith-based youth work courses is the attention many give to exploring theology, values and ethics which many of the more behavioural-based secular courses do not address or address in less depth. For all youth workers it is important to examine their practice if they work for institutions which hold strong convictions. For the faith-based workers there may be pressure on them to gain new members or 'deepen' beliefs of young people. The most pertinent ethical issues relate to the role of the worker, the process of youth work and the desired outcomes of the work.

The role of youth worker is crucial in the ethical debate. The informal education process provides space for young people to explore personal and social issues for their own development. It is important that this working space is held by the youth worker and is not crowded out by the worker's own beliefs or values. If an informal education process is adopted it is appropriate for youth workers to share their own faith, beliefs or values when asked, provided the workers make it clear that the belief is held personally and is one of many options available to the young people. The youth worker as the facilitator of the process works with the young person to explore the issues and options in the widest sense and, if the young person wishes, helps make choices and support change. As the youth worker may be a role model for the young person it is important that the worker explores fairly the range of options available and speaks of his or her own belief choices frankly and openly but without 'closing down' other possibilities for the young person. It is also important that the 'animateur' part of the youth work role is not suppressed by a clinical correctness. One would expect youth workers who accompany young people on outdoor expeditions to share their enthusiasm for the outdoor life. Similarly, it is wholly appropriate for youth workers to share their enthusiasm for their faith in a spirit of offering rather than direction.

The youth work context

The process of youth work is not the same as the content of the work. Although the process should meet the NYA's ethical and professional principles, work can be explicitly religious, or faith based, and still be good youth work. For example, a piece of work may involve young women creating a religious dance for a Hindu ceremony. If the young people are aware and have 'opted in', and if they are involved and not coerced or manipulated, this will enable them to develop, and they will be empowered and educated through the process. Although the content of the work is explicitly religious, the process is informal education and the result can be good-quality youth work. The main ethical issue rests on the awareness of young people within the process and whether they are enabled or disabled in making choices.

The desired outcomes, or aims or objectives, can also indicate whether youth work is in accord with the NYA's ethical and professional principles. If the principal aim of the work with young people is to make new or better members of a religious organisation, then the informal education process will inevitably be contorted. No longer is the work functioning on the agenda of the young people in negotiation with the youth worker, but the worker is working to a specific outcome which is predetermined, and thus the young person will be more likely to be moulded and directed to meet the aim. The pressure will be less empowering and more directive, and will diverge from the informal education model of making informed choices described earlier. The British Council of Churches (1976: 23) makes this point well:

> A religion can only encourage the personal freedom of its young people towards their future if the religion is free with regard to its own future. If Christian faith sought merely to reduplicate itself, to form young Christians who were the exact repetition of the previous generation, to pass on Christian faith as if it were a parcel handed down from generation to generation, then it would be very difficult to distinguish between the passing on of this sort of thing and closed authoritative instruction or even indoctrination.

Faith institutions do not necessarily have narrow or convergent objectives. There is a desire for political and religious awareness and competence in many institutions that can be a primary aim with a secondary wish that a proportion of young people might choose to affiliate with a particular ideology or institution. As Marsh (2006: 12) says of Jewish youth work:

> Informal education methodologies encourage youth workers to engage in conversations with our young people, and enable young people to explore their own identities through a myriad of experiences and dialogues, to set them on their own journeys.

Miller (1990: 258) further elaborates on this theme:

> If we conceive of the locale of religious education as a dynamic, flexible, and forward looking community of learners and teachers, what kinds of goals do we seek?
>
> Rather than outline specific goals in terms of description, what we need are areas in which generalised goals may be established. If we take a pluralistic and flexible view of the meaning of religious maturity, we cannot expect results

in terms of fixed beliefs or codes of behaviour. If we take seriously the meaning of human freedom responding to vague stimuli, both human and divine, we may hope to evoke insights but we cannot determine assembly line results.

Institutions operating more open policies will aim for an ideological maturity among the young people with whom they work. If the institutions also meet the NYA principles this can represent best practice in the field.

Youth work training

Another element that plays a seminal role in the collective understanding of professional ethics is the training and qualification of youth workers. In England, the standards that lay down the level of training and attainment that is sufficient to become a 'qualified youth worker' have largely been determined by the Joint Negotiating Committee and The National Youth Agency in its role of validating courses, based on the National Occupational Standards for Youth Work. Although many youth work courses have been run by colleges which were founded by religious denominations, the courses that have been professionally validated, until recently, have largely been secular, with the religious element implicit and integral rather than explicitly explored. The rise in the need for Christian youth workers has been accompanied by a corresponding rise in Christian youth work courses. There are now a range of colleges which combine youth work with applied theology to equip youth workers for posts within faith contexts as well as for work in secular settings. While most of these courses are Christian, there is now at least one Muslim youth work course in Britain. An issue that arises for many students on these courses is how youth work fits with other work with young people within a religious centre that uses a more directive behavioural style. It is important that the students are able to understand that using a more formal education model can be effective and useful for the young people but differs from youth work. The differences occur in that the focus may be on the desired outcomes (bringing to faith or deepening faith) and that the agenda is set by the organisation. Although it may be argued that young people can be empowered by the outcomes of such training they are not necessarily empowered by the process. A parallel can be made with statutory education where young people are undoubtedly empowered by gaining academic qualifications but do not actively participate in setting the agenda or negotiating the process. This raises an issue for the broader world of youth work where many youth workers are working in multi-agency teams and often to more prescribed agendas. For example, many youth work organisations receive funding by specifying outcomes for the work which can have implications for how it is delivered. Youth workers need to be able to examine the process and see whether the amount of direction and potential coercion is in line with the broader professional ethics.

Ethical issues for youth workers

There are ethical issues that youth workers encounter personally when being employed by an organisation that is in existence because of the belief system it expounds. There are questions about the extent to which youth workers' personal faith corresponds to that of the organisation and how, where there are differences, the situation is resolved.

Many working in faith-based youth work are drawn in with a strong sense of vocation and with strong ideological aims. The worker may have a powerful personal need to 'share the story' and this may impair the central experiential element of informal education through youth work. It may be that such a worker would be more comfortable with a delivered formal education approach, and much religious instruction is delivered using more directive practice. In some faiths this is part of a process of traditional dissemination and there is an understanding of the strengths and weaknesses of this sort of delivery. Nesbitt and Jackson's (1994) work with Hindu and Sikh children shows a range of formal and informal methods employed (Nesbitt 1993). It is important for there to be clarity about what process is being used and that a more directive training approach is not seen as youth work. The strength of the youth work process in spiritual development is important, and open, participative ways of working are to be encouraged. When youth work is being established, questions that may be asked (based on the NYA principles) include:

- Are young people treated with respect and individually valued?
- Are young people's rights respected and promoted, and are they able to make their own decisions?
- Is the organisation providing a safe place for young people and are they learning through challenging educational activities?
- Does the project promote social justice for young people and society by encouraging respect for difference and diversity, and do youth workers challenge discrimination?
- Is the project run with professional integrity?

As a group of practitioners with a commitment and investment in youth work as a 'profession', it is entirely appropriate and responsible for us to ask these questions of each other's practice, both formally and informally, regardless of faith, or ideological position.

For those youth workers who wish to use professional youth work methods there may be difficulty where individual young people make choices which conflict with personally held values. An example may be a young person choosing to have an abortion where the youth worker's principles are against this. It is important in this situation that if the youth worker cannot enable the young person to explore a range of choices, then the worker should make this clear and allow the young person to decide whether the worker is the most appropriate person to help. What matters most is that there is an integrity in the relationship and, just as doctors may declare a personal position that alters the consultation, so may youth workers make similar declarations. Other youth workers may put increased value on the youth work process rather than on the outcome and are able to suspend their own judgement and preference, allowing the young person to make an informed choice. In this situation it is important for youth workers to realise the impossibility of being 'totally objective' but to endeavour to be aware of the impact of their own value systems on the process. However youth workers deal with this, it is important that the matter is taken up in supervision so that there can be good exploration of the effect of managing a difficult issue and workers can resolve any internal issues to free up their future work.

Another key area for youth workers to address is their awareness of the vulnerability of young people as they search for meaning, identity and a sense of belonging. This is especially important for those youth workers whose values reflect such concepts as salvation, damnation, redemption or reincarnation. These concepts are very powerful and have to be used sensitively so that young people retain control and power over their own lives.

Conclusion

It is very easy to point a finger from a secular youth work position at faith institutions and be convinced of poor or partial practice. It is important to note, though, that the youth service was born out of the conscience of individuals with faith and faith groups, and much of the emphasis within youth work on social justice has its roots in the campaigning and service of nineteeth-century faith activists.

All youth workers have a value system that informs their work, and effective dialogue between youth work practitioners of all ideological, religious or political persuasions can only be beneficial in the development of 'professional' ethics. It is apparent that the discussion of ethics and youth work needs to be a more collective exercise to sharpen the focus and confidence of youth work practitioners. There are several principles that are central to any ethical debate on work with young people, especially when the work occurs from a particular ideological perspective, be that religious, political or single-issue groups. These are as follows:

- It is ethically sound for organisations to share their perspectives, skills, knowledge and values. It is not only sound but it is irresponsible of organisations to withhold collective knowledge and traditions that belong to everyone in society regardless of age.
- Young people have a right to develop spiritually and politically as well as mentally, physically and socially. It is not enough to leave this development to

haphazard processes but there should be an understanding of the process of how people develop frameworks of thought and living, and this should form part of the youth work curriculum. Secular youth work should examine the degree to which the religious and political development of young people is addressed in the curriculum and make appropriate provision for this.

- Youth work is a means to empower young people politically and religiously. By having an understanding of established ideological frameworks, young people are able to use these and be enabled by them, and are also able to be critically reflective of groups abusing the youth work process for institutional gain.
- Qualified youth work practitioners should feel confident to challenge ideologically based youth work using the nationally accepted statements of purpose and other sets of ethical principles developed collectively through training and debate.
- Through this increased confidence in practice youth workers should feel able to challenge and resist unprofessional work that disempowers young people, especially that work which exploits the adolescent search for identity, belonging and meaning.
- Faith organisations should be encouraged to continue to examine their work with young people and to use best professional practice. This enables their youth workers to work with young people to facilitate growth and development while offering information about the organisation.

Active dialogue among youth workers with the whole range of ideological, political and faith viewpoints can only challenge and sharpen the professional edge and ethics of youth work.

Questions for reflection and discussion

1   Can a youth worker combine more formal ways of working with young people, for example religious instruction, with their usual youth work methods? If they do, what sorts of issues might arise for them and the young people?
2   How might a youth worker who is attached to a faith-based organisation work with young people to challenge the influence of fundamentalist indoctrination?
3   How could you challenge a faith-based organisation to use nationally accepted statements of purpose and ethical principles to assess and critique its work with young people? What barriers might you have to overcome and how would you go about this?

Recommended reading

Green, M. (2006) *A Journey of Discovery: Spirituality and Spiritual Development in Youth Work*, Leicester: The National Youth Agency. This is a report commissioned by the Department for Education and Skills, which builds on a consultation exercise to help form a collective understanding of spiritual development in youth work.

Youth and Policy No. 92 (Summer 2006). This is a special issue on Muslim youth work comprising a collection of interesting articles which explore some critical issues relating to youth work in Muslim and Jewish settings.

References

Ahmed, S., Banks, S. and Duce, C. (2007) *Walking Alongside Young People: Challenges and Opportunities for Faith Communities*, Durham: Durham University and Churches' Regional Commission in the North East.

Banks, S. (1996) 'Youth work, informal education and professionalisation: the issues in the 1990s', *Youth and Policy*, 54: 13–25.

Banks, S. (2009) 'Values and ethics in work with young people', in J. Wood and J. Hine (eds) *Work with Young People: Developments in Theory, Policy and Practice*, London: Sage.

British Council of Churches (1976) *Child and the Church*, London: CGMC.

Church of England (1991) *How Faith Grows*, London: National Society/Church Housing Publishing.

Church of England (1996) *Youth A Part*, London: Church House Publishing.

Freud, S. (1927) *Future of an Illusion*, London: Penguin.

Green, M.J. (1997) 'A religious perspective for youth work', in N. Kendra and I. Ledgerwood (eds) *The Challenge for the Future: Towards the New Millennium for the Youth Service*, Lyme Regis: Russell House.

Hamid, S. (2006) 'Models of Muslim youthwork: between reform and empowerment', *Youth and Policy*, 92: 81–90.

HMSO (1969) *Youth and Community Work in the 70s*, London: HMSO.

Keesing, R. (1969) *Cultural Anthropology*, Orlando: Holt, Rinehart & Winston.

Marsh, S. (2006) 'Exploring the development of Jewish identity in young people', *Youth and Policy*, 92: 47–57.

Marx, K. (1938) *Capital*, London: George Allen & Unwin.

Miller, R. (1990) 'Theology and the future of religious education', in L. Francis and A. Thatcher (eds) *Christian Perspectives for Education*, Leominster: Gracewing.

National Youth Agency (2004) *Ethical Conduct in Youth Work: A Statement of Values and Principles from the National Youth Agency*, Leicester: The National Youth Agency.

Nesbitt, E. (1993) 'The transmission of Christian tradition in an ethically diverse society', in R. Barot (ed.) *Religion and Ethnicity: Minorities and Social Change in the Metropolis*, Kampen Netherlands: Kok Pharos.

Nesbitt, E. and Jackson, R. (1994) 'Aspects of cultural transmission in a diaspora Sikh community', *Journal of Sikh Studies*, 18, 1: 55–67.

Rose, D. (2005) 'The world of the Jewish youth movement', *The Encyclopedia of Informal Education*, www.infed.org/informaljewisheducation/jewish_youth_movements.htm (accessed July 2009).

Wallace, A. (1972) *The Death and Rebirth of the Seneca*, New York: Vintage.

<table>
<tr><td>9</td></tr>
</table>

Youth workers as critical interpreters and mediators

Ethical issues in working with black young people

Umme F. Imam and Rick Bowler

Introduction

This chapter explores the complexities that arise in working with black[1] young people in Western contexts and the ethical issues facing black and white[2] practitioners as they fulfil their professional responsibilities in educating and supporting black young people to negotiate racism in everyday life. All youth workers mediate and negotiate within and between structures of power, influence and authority in their roles as informal educators. However, those working with black young people mediate between distinctive and unequal systems and structures that arise through racism and inequality.

The analysis in this chapter is undertaken on two levels. The first addresses issues that are significant for all workers, focusing on the primacy of Western values, the normativity of whiteness and the implications for black and white workers in their work with young people from minority communities. The second focuses on the dilemmas and issues faced by black workers, with specific reference to work with young people of South Asian[3] origin. Examples drawn from interviews and discussions with workers and young people are used to illustrate ethical issues in practice. Our conclusion synthesises the discussion and identifies ways in which black and white professionals can position themselves to move away from promoting ethnocentric values to more egalitarian practice.

Recent trends in policy and theory

In the past decade, the landscape for race relations and race equality has changed rapidly and dramatically in Britain (Sallah and Howson 2007). A key incident was the racist murder of a young man, Stephen Lawrence, in London in 1993 (Macpherson 1999). Following this murder the influence of institutional racism within public services (specifically the police) was acknowledged and important statutory responsibilities were placed on all public bodies to promote race equality (OPSI 2009). However, the focus quickly shifted to strategies for developing 'community cohesion' following episodes of violence between white and Asian communities in various parts of the country in 2001, further intensified after the London bombings of 2005. These events provided the opportunity to shift from a fraught racial equality approach to a more comfortable community cohesion and integration strategy, which could pass responsibility for difficulties and problems back to black communities (Davies 2008).

These events also led a range of political commentators on the Left and Right to express the view that multiculturalism has failed and/or it is to blame for the lack of cohesion in society. A further factor in the subordinating of these new 'race'-related policy initiatives was the governmental security agenda following the events of 11 September 2001 in USA, the 'War on Terror' and the London bombings in 2005, which led to policies and programmes under the 'Preventing Violent Extremism' (PVE) agenda. PVE goes beyond the aims of community cohesion and integration by adding a focus on identifying potential religious extremists. In his critical considerations on youth work and anti-racist practice, Thomas (2009: 283) asserts that 'PVE is neither making a helpful contribution to community cohesion, or effectively engaging with the political and doctrinal understandings that are attracting a small minority of young Muslims towards extremism'. Predictably and significantly the black youth response to these changes has been an accentuated self-definition on grounds of faith – in rejection of the state-imposed differentiation based on ethnic origin. The emergence of Muslim youth work (Khan 2006) has been a consequence of the racism and alienation faced by black young people and the demonisation of Islam in the Western popular press.

What is clear is that racism continues. Popular racist nationalism has become mainstreamed with the 2009 election victory of two 'fascist' British National Party (BNP) Members of the European Parliament and racist campaigns organised under the umbrella of the so-called 'English Defence League'. The reality for black communities has been an increase in unsafe spaces with a more dangerous and difficult terrain for black young people. Sivananadan (2007: 48) clarifies the connections of these dominant popular and 'newer' forms of racism:

> on the ground a racism that cannot tell a settler from an immigrant, an asylum seeker from a Muslim, a Muslim from a terrorist. All of us non-whites, at first sight, are terrorists or illegals. We wear our passports on our face.

In seeking to understand the complex dynamics of racism, two emerging areas of theory and practice have informed our thinking: critical studies of whiteness (Bonnett 2000; Garner 2007) and critical race theory (Delgado and Stefanic 2001; Gillborn 2008; Taylor *et al.* 2009). In both these fields of study, whiteness is critically examined as the place and space of dominance where privilege is masked through the powers of normativity. The normative culture of 'whiteworld' (Gillborn 2008) utilises a range of trickery to hide the depths and levels of racism in order to appear as the place from which universal values of equity and justice are born. Critical race theory and critical theories on racism suggest that the normative 'whiteworld' culture holds deep veins of racism embedded in institutions, cultural production and in and around individual relations. These invasive and evasive ways of knowing hide their own logic through the process of racialisation. Racialisation produces and reproduces racist logic that individualises and naturalises 'race' (Miles 1989). In Western societies, it is the difference of the 'other' that signifies the arrival of 'race' and the cause of racist sentiment. The historical realities of racism, the material disadvantages that are structured into society and the symbolic racial markers sustained within dominant white culture are overlooked or denied. In 'whiteworld' it may be seen that there is a two-faced approach to being, becoming and belonging. Entry is possible but belonging is always contingent upon some often hidden and always racialised rules about what it is to be British.

As mentioned earlier, in Britain, at least two main policy agendas can be identified. On the one hand there is the developing equalities and human rights agenda that speaks to inclusion, integration and diversity. On the other hand there are the structural border controls that mark out the sub-citizen, incarcerate the asylum seeker, including children and young people, and survey the Muslim and all who 'look Muslim'. These two faces have unfolded within the persistence of a dominant story that feeds a symbolic racist discourse offering a white imagery on being, becoming and belonging. Thus much of the resentment about poor services and changing worlds is attributed by 'poor whites' to black people coded as 'the foreigner', 'the Muslim', 'the immigrant', 'the other' (Garner *et al.* 2009). This national racist mythology is underpinned by white supremacist imagery that feeds into loss and victimhood, where white people can blame black people for the predicament in which they find themselves. Described as postcolonial melancholia (Gilroy 2004), this perpetuation of racist form persists due to the lack of political leadership and a serious gap in anti-racism within the formal and public education sectors. This racist logic also leaves a gaping hole into which black young people fall and from which they learn the negative and dangerous responses to the ongoing exclusions and violations they experience.

Racism is embedded in everyday life (Bhavnani *et al.* 2006). In dominant discourse racism has been silenced by the incorporation of the terms of diversity. In dominant discourse racism has been individualised as if it were 'natural' and its history and deep embeddedness in the national state structures and transnational systems of power are denied. 'Race', ethnicity and culture are reduced as if they are the same (Gunaratnam 2003). The historical realities of racism, the material disadvantages that are structured into society and the symbolic racial markers sustained within dominant white culture are denied.

Youth work in a plural society

A key element of the youth worker's role is to support the self-emancipation of young people through promoting understanding of how the ideologies and values of the majority influence and limit their lives, inhibiting participation and equality. Work with black young people needs to be focused on helping them to understand, challenge and cope with the demands of the multiple cultural systems they inhabit. The situation would be complex in itself without the addition of racism and cultural oppression to the dynamics, and their influence on individuals and how they conceive of themselves.

Two critical factors complicate work for practitioners negotiating different racial terrains and understanding the multiple cultural contexts that black young people inhabit in a postcolonial world (Mama 1995). The first is the normative supremacy and implicit universalism of the majority Western/white culture, ethics and values, and the subordination of minority cultures and identities. Second, complexities arise through the interface of individualist and collectivist philosophical traditions and values, not just between one culture and another, but between 'whiteworld' and the multiplicities of all of the rest of 'others'.

The hegemony of Western values

Youth work does not take place in a vacuum, nor do youth workers hold neutral principles and values. Both are subject to cultural and societal influences which impact upon the work and workers. In a culturally diverse society it is expected that there should be a heterogeneity of cultures, traditions, ethics and values, which are fluid and dynamic and interact and intersect to form new configurations and positions (Woolett *et al.* 1994). However, despite pluralism in society, the superiority of the majority values prevails because 'the normative grid that locates cultural diversity at the same time serves to contain cultural difference: the universalism that paradoxically permits diversity masks ethnocentric norms' (Maclaren 1995: 213–214).

Consequently, in their work with black young people workers find themselves negotiating a two-tier value system. The differential occurs because despite the pluralism in British society, the values of the majority are presented as universal and progressive and those of minorities as inferior and regressive. The inequality is further confirmed by assumptions that minority cultures are fixed and static and their movement from one ethnic context to another has involved a single cultural change through adaptation to the new situation and in relation to the majority, rather than the fluid and continuous change attributed to majority cultures (Woolett *et al.* 1994).

In exploring youth work within a plural society, whiteness and issues of dominance are beginning to be put under closer interrogation (Webb 2001; Sallah and Howson 2007). Dominant 'whiteworld' constructions attempt to naturalise, essentialise and minoritise 'other' cultures. This leaves whiteness to occupy the place of the norm from which it can mark the 'other'. This homogenising of culture appears to black and white young people as normative. In the absence of alternative experiences, possibilities and narratives this norm of whiteness can become desired. Whiteness therefore needs to be problematised by youth workers if white and black young people are to be helped to critically locate their positions in and resistance to it.

Critical professionals must develop counter-racist narratives that accurately interpret the racism in 'whiteworld' and mediate with young people the journeys that can build critical consciousness and critical compassion. Critical interpretation needs critical literacy. This is essential in supporting black young people to develop their 'resilience to racisms' and critical understanding of culture through engaging in an active interpretation of how to locate and counter racist environments. How practitioners and educators engage young people in these processes and develop 'critical literacy on countering racisms' must be a core concern of professional practice. Workers cannot claim to be conducting ethical practice unless they build links between critical literacy and cultural competence while maintaining the focus on raising aspiration (Ladson-Billings 2001). These are the cornerstones of work with all young people.

Ethical issues faced by black workers working with young people of South Asian heritage

In light of the preceding discussion on the dominance of Western values, we cannot assume a common or neutral ethical framework which may be of relevance to practitioners working with all constituencies of young people growing up in Britain. Practitioner ethics are socially constructed and reflect dominant norms; social and institutional structures will inevitably define and normalise ethics in any area of work. Banks (2004: 222–223) suggests that the ethical dilemmas commonly encountered in the welfare professions fall into three main categories: conflicts between the self-determination (autonomy) of service users and what the professional considers to be in their best interests; conflicts between the rights and welfare of different people; and conflicting value systems.

In the context of work with minority ethnic communities, the dilemmas faced are made more complex by the fact that these communities may not share the values arising from Western individualistic thinking. Practitioners working with black young people face additional ethical challenges deriving from the different and unequal value systems of workers, agencies, communities and young people. In practice this is significant in two ways. First, there is the assumption of majority values and norms, particularly those relating to individualism. Little attention may be given to the complexity of young people's lives and the continuous drawing and redrawing of boundaries as they negotiate different cultural contexts and changing social and cultural landscapes. Second, issues arise due to conflicting values of workers and the agencies and institutions which recruit and employ them.

Self-determination, rights and culture

Central to youth work practice is the principle of self-determination, the non-directive enabling of young people to make decisions and choices in their lives leading to self-emancipation (Smith 1988). The concept of self-determination has come from rights-based approaches to moral thought which are rooted in Western liberal traditions and philosophies. In particular, the right to self-determination is firmly established in Kantian principles and the recognition that individuals should have autonomy in making their own choices and decisions (Banks 2006). It has been widely interpreted, ranging from the absolute right of individuals to do as they please to intervention by practitioners based on their beliefs about what is in the best interests of the individual. In youth work practice, despite a parentalist approach, the emphasis has been on promoting self-determination through personal and social education. This has reflected the majority individualistic values with little consideration given to the fact that interdependence rather than independence is the cultural particularity for black young people, and freedom of choice is circumscribed by emotional interdependence and responsibility to family and community (Ahmad 1990: 14).

Practitioners are faced with difficult choices when self-determination by the young person results in conflict with family expectations and interdependence. Another problem with individualist (Kantian) approaches is that when there is conflict between the rights of two individuals, for example, parent and young person, how do we decide whose right to self-determination should prevail? In the case of conflict between the individual and family, mediation between the two generations involves more than just the issues around age and generation. It also involves work between different configurations of cultural systems: the mono-cultural perspectives or the 'old ethnicities' of some parents and the 'new ethnicities' of the young people (Hall 1992).

Case study 9.1 (opposite) illustrates this conflict between the demands, desires and attitudes of parents and offspring.

A female youth worker of Indian origin working in an Asian women's project in a British city was approached by a member whose daughter Asha (aged 18) attended the young women's group. The mother was of Bangladeshi origin and had been in Britain for thirty years. Her husband had died ten years before. The mother was concerned about her daughter's behaviour as she was going out with a white boyfriend and seen to be 'behaving inappropriately' in community settings. This had provoked great censure within the community as she was seen to be too 'Westernised and moving out of her culture'. As a widowed single parent the mother was quite distressed about her daughter's behaviour and the implications this would have for her own honour and respect, as well as that of her other daughters within the community. She asked the youth worker to use her influence to dissuade the young woman from seeing her white boyfriend. Asha had also discussed the situation with the worker. She seemed to be quite serious about the relationship and felt that she should have the right to make her own decision about her future partner and did not really care what the community thought of her.

In discussing and analysing the situation and her own intervention, the worker said she recognised the pressures on the mother from the local community and empathised with her. She also recognised that the young woman was expressing dominant individualistic values into which she had been socialised. The differences in perspectives were inevitable, as they had developed through different social and cultural experiences in South Asia and in Britain. The worker demonstrated her 'epistemic advantage' (Narayan 1989) through her knowledge and understanding of both perspectives. Her task was to work individually, interpreting, translating and mediating between different understandings, experiences and expectations and to help each appreciate the other's perspective. Through discussion in the girls' group and individually, the worker was able to help the young woman appreciate how minority cultures become insular and inflexible as they struggle to preserve cultural traditions in a hostile environment. With the mother, the worker raised awareness that cultural traditions were subject to change and ways in which patriarchal systems work to control women's behaviour. The worker also drew on her own family and their influence in the community to solicit support for the mother and daughter and to acknowledge the inappropriateness of monocultural values and behavioural expectations in a multi-racial setting. The outcome of the intervention was that the mother accepted her daughter's choice and agreed that the young people could get married if they were serious about each other – after they had completed their undergraduate studies. The young woman agreed to modify her behaviour within community settings to save her mother distress and humiliation.

This example highlights the difficulties workers face in mediating between different cultural systems. On the one hand, there is a minority community with its distinctive religious and cultural beliefs and prescribed norms of behaviour. However, this exists and is situated within a majority, where individual rights are paramount and the norms of behaviour are quite different. This does not mean that the worker should collude with harmful cultural traditions, but it requires her to acknowledge the differences between generations which arise out of different cultural values. Some young people may choose to identify with the dominant value system without considering the implications that this may have for them and their situation within minority collectivist traditions. They may not have a good understanding of the complex dynamics of the various influences that shape and mould their thoughts and actions. Intervention in such situations needs to focus on interpreting the relative significance of different social systems in the individual's life and facilitating informed decisions.

Some workers may well perceive this to be a matter of individual choice and the right of the young woman to choose her partner. This would be to view the situation entirely from an individualistic perspective, and they would not be enabling her to make well-informed decisions. The young woman would be at risk of being isolated and ostracised, first, because she would be seen to be flouting religious and cultural values, and second, through being 'black' in 'whiteworld'. The consequences for the entire family would be equally damaging as they would be held responsible for her behaviour and also face rejection and isolation. She herself would be alienated from support systems which provide refuge from the racism of wider society.

For practitioners, the issue is how to promote individual choice at the same time as acknowledging pluralism in cultures and the constraints on the individual. The task for the worker would be to support the mother and the family within the community to challenge the patriarchal systems which control women through notions of respectability and honour. Intervention should also be informed by an understanding of why minority cultures appear to resist change and protect traditional values. As Kishwar (1996: 12) explains, minority communities in the West have become more culturally inflexible than those in South Asia because they are threatened by Westernisation and loss of identity. Ejaz (1991), exploring the concept of self-determination and intervention by practitioners within the Indian context, suggests that due to the collectivist cultural value of interdependence, service users are not threatened by the 'spirit of dependency' and are 'socially open to advice and guidance from others', especially from someone who has greater knowledge either through education or through age and experience. Black workers report that this is an important factor when negotiating support for young people with parents, and is not construed as interference in personal affairs.

Youth workers are often faced with dilemmas relating to balancing the needs, interests and rights of one individual against those of other people. In resolving such dilemmas the utilitarian premise that the right action is the one that promotes the greatest good for the greatest number is often invoked (Banks 2006). In the preceding example, such an approach might have entailed disregarding Asha's feelings and prioritising the welfare of her mother and sisters over her own. It is evident that there are no easy solutions to such ethical dilemmas and often workers are left with having to make choices between equally undesirable outcomes and to cope with the residue after making a difficult decision (see Chapter 1 for a discussion of this feature of dilemmas).

Accountability, loyalty and the dominance of the white agenda

The employment of black workers in mainstream and black-led agencies also raises distinctive issues of accountability and loyalty: to young people, communities and employers. In black-led projects, including faith-based work, conflicts often arise between the personal/professional values of workers and the traditional values of the employers.

The development of youth work and recruitment of black workers raises issues of ethics in the actions taken and the discriminatory effects of practices adopted to counter discrimination. On the one hand, some local authorities and other agencies have adopted a radical approach, taking positive action through training and apprenticeship schemes specifically targeting black trainees and workers. As a result, qualified black workers have been recruited with the experience, knowledge, values and skills to work effectively with black young people. Like their counterparts in social work practice, the workers who come in with knowledge, skills, experience and 'a commitment to fight racism unreservedly' (Patel 1995: 33) may find themselves to be marginalised by the agency and other colleagues (including black colleagues) as they are seen as 'too black', 'not objective', 'unprofessional' and 'too close to the black community'. The vulnerability of such workers is further heightened by the fact that other black workers may be used against them.

A second approach, based in liberal multiculturalism, is reflected by agencies that simply absolve themselves of the responsibility to meet the needs of black young people by appointing black people as youth workers. The ethnicity or 'race' of the worker – being black or Bangladeshi – becomes the qualification for working with black young people and gives them the credentials for practice. In the words of one worker, he was appointed on the 'ticket of culture'. Black workers who do survive in mainstream organisations which take the liberal multicultural approach do so through their commitment to personal and professional development, and not through the responsibility of their employers to staff development and training.

However, as Patel comments, not all black workers act 'in the best interests of racial and social justice, or for the greater good' (Patel 1995: 33). For some black workers, appointed as a result of liberal policies, 'equal opportunities' become 'equal opportunism'. Such workers reflect individualistic values and are committed only to themselves and their professional advancement. They feel accountable solely to their employers and not to young people or communities. In their professional practice they adopt either a 'traditionalist' or 'Western' approach corresponding to employer expectations. In the case of the former, they justify their employment by demonstrating stereotypical traditional values which are completely at odds with those of young people. Those employed because they are seen to be 'Westernised' and 'progressive' use their professional platform to deny ethnicity and difference, and ignore the impact of these issues on black young people by adopting and advocating the values of the institutions and agencies uncritically. Such practices and outcomes demonstrate how inequality and oppression are reinforced and confirmed by the very strategies used to counter and challenge discrimination and disadvantage (Ben-Tovim et al. 1992).

One of the main reasons for appointing black workers is to form 'a bridge between white-dominated institutions and black young people' (Patten 1997: 29). The strengths of black workers are seen as their ability to identify with issues faced by black young people; to serve as good role models; and to use their skills and experience to empower young people. This position, despite being one of strength, is also one of vulnerability. As they mediate between the unequal black and white systems and people, this position is in itself precarious. They can be perceived to be 'too close to black communities' by employers who question their loyalty and professionalism. On the other hand, they may also be regarded as 'too close to white institutions' and their loyalty to black communities and young people may also be questioned. Furthermore, the absence of ethical considerations in their recruitment and support confirms the dominance and normativity of 'whiteworld'. Case study 9.2 illustrates some of the problems faced by a newly employed black worker and illustrates how privilege is masked through the powers of normativity. It reveals the lack of critical literacy and understanding of racism by a white manager considered to be an 'exemplar practitioner'.

Case study 9.2

A recently qualified black youth worker was recruited by an integrated youth project to support its movement from being a predominantly 'white project' to 'integrating' black young people. The project was widely regarded as 'cutting edge' – that is, at the forefront of good practice. The project users were predominantly white, working-class males. No significant work had been undertaken to prepare the black or white young people, the workers or the organisation for the new developments.

Within a very short period of time at the project the black worker observed and encountered repeated incidents of verbal abuse and threats. These experiences were encountered in the immediate vicinity outside the centre. The black worker became acutely aware that these racist incidents were not understood by all his white colleagues. The offending white males were users of the project. They had learnt to 'police' their racist language when around white professionals. The black worker sought help from his manager about managing these 'in and around work' racial aggressions. He hoped his experienced manager could suggest strategies for managing the added stress associated with being black, the racial 'other' in and around the work. The manager told him a story about how community and youth work can be stressful. 'It's the same for everyone' appeared to be the wisdom. The manager's own response for dealing with this 'in and around work' stress was to 'chill out' at home and 'to put work out of your mind' when away from it. The black worker realised in that moment that the white project manager – 'the exemplar anti-racist practitioner' – had no real or critical understanding of the power and impact of everyday racism nor of his collusion with the everyday racial micro-aggressions which black people experience in 'whiteworld'.

The project manager described in this account had probably never really considered his own position of privilege within the racist environments in which he and his colleagues lived and worked. His lack of awareness and 'dysconsciousness' or 'distorted way of thinking' (King 2006: 73) reproduced an additional racial micro-aggression (Sue *et al.* 2008, 2009), adding to the negative impact on the black worker and by implication black young people. The project manager's dysconsciousness seems to have created a block to any critical thinking about the induction process and the need for culturally competent assessment tools when considering the black worker's ability to succeed in the job. The account presented here suggests that the white project manager had never critically engaged with 'whiteness' and therefore viewed racism as only embodied within the local 'overtly ignorant white lives' of some adults and young people in the neighbourhood. These moments of overt racist behaviours need to be critically located so that project managers are able to comprehend that 'other lives' embody 'other realities' and that these are racialised. It is vital that critical and systematic work is undertaken with the white young people in neighbourhoods to address how their own situations and knowledge related to whiteness leave them unprepared for 'integration' with black young people. This example illuminates some of the ethical issues that arise when white youth work operates without a critical lens on whiteness.

Integration versus segregation

Contradictory policy developments provide further complications to the work undertaken with South Asian young people. First, the emphasis on the integration of minorities and their cohesion with the majority mitigates against work with specific ethnic groups. Second, the PVE agenda and promotion of work with Muslim youth instigates separation and segregation within multi-faith South Asian communities. Youth workers who are on the front line of engagement with communities and young people report frustration and discontent from majority and minority communities owing to 'preferential treatment' for Muslims and 'discrimination' against non-Muslims. Practitioners working with Muslim youth also struggle with the dichotomies and tensions between working with young people in an Islamic way or working with diverse Muslim youth, and between proselytising or empowerment (Hamid 2006; Hussain 2006). The ethical predicament for practitioners is further compounded by the fact that young people are increasingly asserting Muslim identities as a way of resisting the limitations imposed by hegemonic definitions of ethnic identity (Malik 2006).

Practitioners are also faced with choices and dilemmas in undertaking single sex work, particularly with South Asian girls and young women. They find themselves juggling religious and cultural constraints on work with South Asian young women with the competing demands of secular provision, which addresses diversity and difference and does not homogenise this group of young people. Indeed, diversity and differentiation among South Asian young people, not just on grounds of gender but, in relation to country of origin, ethnicity, faith, pattern of migration to the UK, rural/urban origins and sexual orientation require black and white practitioners to recognise the partiality of their own experiences and knowledge for working effectively with different constituencies of young people.

Multiple roles and expectations

Ethical dilemmas are also presented by the multiple roles that workers occupy (Banks 2004). Collectivist values compound these dilemmas further through different role expectations – by young people, by communities, other workers and other communities. Conflicts occur when these different roles as professional practitioners and as members of particular communities are brought to play in a specific situation. The case of Asha (Case study 9.1) is a good example of the complexity of the position which black workers face. Case study 9.3 is based on an account from another female black worker living and working in a predominantly South Asian neighbourhood.

Case study 9.3

I was working with a young woman who was going out with a married man from our community. The man's wife knew that I was a youth worker and approached me for help. I was already working with the young woman who was a regular member of the girls' group. As a member of the community I knew about the man's reputation and that he was abusing the young woman as well as his wife . . . it was a nightmare . . . made worse when he threatened me and other members of my family about interfering in his personal affairs.

This worker is caught up in an extremely difficult situation. As a youth work practitioner she has to work with issues of autonomy and self-determination as well as her professional assessment of the young woman's welfare. As a member of a particular community and a practitioner working within that community she is known to all the parties concerned, who have their own perceptions and expectations of her different roles. This also heightens her vulnerability as a practitioner in bringing together the personal and professional roles. Such situations are not uncommon, where issues of loyalty and accountability to the community are brought into play alongside professional roles and responsibilities (as described by Sercombe in Chapter 5). In resolving these issues workers have to assess critically their roles in relation to the community and their profession and justify their approaches in the light of their personal and professional ethics and values. The guidance given at the end of Chapter 5 is very helpful in this respect.

Conclusion: moving beyond ethnocentric values and ethics

Youth workers who work with diverse constituencies of young people cannot assume universalistic perspectives that homogenise differences and confirm the dominance of majority norms. Practitioners need to move beyond simplistic explanations that polarise Western and non-Western, black and white, traditional and Westernised, individualist and collectivist, and provide the space for fusion and complication between these in acknowledgement and validation of the complexity and diversity of young people's lives. Mark Smith, in initiating the discussion on the ethics underpinning work with young people in a multi-ethnic context, suggests that the central task for youth workers is to enable young people to develop the ability to think critically in order to:

address their own culture, to own their own experiences, and hence to speak in their own voices . . . people must also learn what is good, they must learn what values are central to human life and well being and how such values are transmitted and distorted in the interests of the powerful. Finally, people must learn about the structural and ideological forces which influence and restrict their lives.

(Smith 1988: 114)

The task of the youth worker, therefore, is to facilitate the process through which young people are able critically to evaluate and identify the values that are fundamental to their welfare. What is important, then, is the ability of workers to move between different social and cultural systems, to relate to different constituencies of people: black and white, disabled and able-bodied, lesbian, gay, bisexual and heterosexual, women and men, and across different social classes. In other words, they have to become what Giroux (1994: 167–168) has termed 'border crossers':

educators have to become more than intellectual tourists. We must move into the spheres, where we take up different contexts, geographies, different languages, of otherness and recognise the otherness in ourselves . . . we also have to recognise the partiality of our views.

The acknowledgement of the partiality of different experiences and views is crucial to this process. Such an acknowledgement may be problematic from majorities, who through their dominance have pushed minorities into occupying such a position. The case studies cited earlier illustrate how black workers have usually worked from this basic premise, recognising the partiality of their understandings and values in relation to those of black and white young people and communities. Patricia Hill Collins (1990: 236) suggests that this positioning may be possible when 'partiality and not universality is the condition of being heard'. The purpose of youth work – to promote the self-determination and self-emancipation of young people through collective action – provides the opportunity for this condition to be imposed upon all people who come together with this objective. In advocating this positioning we can draw from the work of black feminists who have attempted to address issues of essentialism and universalism in women's groups. Nira Yuval Davies (1994) proposes the notion of *transversalism* as distinct from universalism, based on such a partial positioning. It is based on two related concepts of 'rooting' and 'shifting': each individual is rooted in her own identity and culture and shifts in order to put herself in the position of the other.

With reference to an inclusive framework for ethics and values in youth work, we can propose transversal values and ethics which are of relevance to all groups of young people. Practitioners may be rooted in their own perspectives and values but shift in order to place themselves in the position of the service user or young person with different values. What is important is that in shifting one does not lose one's own rooting and values:

> All people can learn to centre in another experience, validate it, judge it by its own standards without need of comparison or need to adopt the framework as their own . . . one has no need to de-centre anyone in order to centre someone else.
>
> (Brown 1989, quoted in Yuval-Davis 1994: 193)

Moving beyond ethnocentric values requires this partial positioning from all groups that come together for collective action – majorities and minorities. This is learning that white people will have to derive from the experiences of people whose perspectives and values they have historically decentred and denied.

Questions for reflection and discussion

1   What are the ethical issues for critical black and white youth workers in supporting black young people in developing their resilience to racism?

2   Why is it important for white workers to become 'border crossers' in undertaking youth work with black young people? How is this illustrated in Case study 9.1 about the young Asian woman with a white boyfriend?

3   Why is it important for all workers to acknowledge the partiality of their own knowledge and values? Are the concepts of 'rooting' and 'shifting' as described in the conclusion to this chapter helpful in promoting more egalitarian values and practice? ('Each individual is rooted in her own identity and culture and shifts in order to put herself in the position of the other'.)

Recommended reading

Garner, S. (2007) *Whiteness: An Introduction,* London: Routledge. This book offers the reader an excellent introduction to the study of whiteness. Garner explores the privilege and power of whiteness and introduces the reader to the key European and American arguments on the subject. Garner identifies that the focus on challenging racism is essential in any critical study of whiteness.

Ladson-Billings, G. and Gillborn, D. (eds) (2006) *The Routledge Falmer Reader in Multicultural Education,* London: RoutledgeFalmer. This critical reader in multicultural education explores theories and concepts on 'race' and racism and helpfully relates these to identities, practices and methods. The book covers work from Britain and the USA that has relevance to community and youth work policy-makers, managers, researchers and practitioners.

Sallah, M. and Howson, C. (eds) (2007) *Working with Black Young People*, Lyme Regis: Russell House Publishing. Sallah and Howson have edited a detailed and exemplary overview of the salient arguments and issues relevant to work with all young people through the lens of working with black young people.

Notes

1 We use the term 'black' to refer to people who share common experiences of racism and colonisation in Britain. This usage has been contested on grounds of denying ethnicity and cultural identity. In youth work practice, however, in the absence of a more widely acceptable term, practitioners and young people continue to use the term and increasingly reject ethnicity in favour of religion as the signifier of their identity. The term 'black' is used here because it continues to be 'a source of unified strength and solidarity opening up more opportunities for celebrating and affirming ethnic identity' (Ahmad 1990: 2–3).

2 The term 'white' is used to signify the privilege and power of the dominant majority in Western societies. It should be understood in the political context of whiteworld and 'whiteness' where whiteness is viewed as both a racial discourse and a privileging location (Leonardo 2006; Garner 2007).

3 'South Asian' is used to refer to people of Bangladeshi, Indian and Pakistani heritage who share common origins in the Indian subcontinent, a heritage of collectivist cultures and the experience of 'cultural racism' in Britain (Ahmed 1986).

References

Ahmed, S. (1986) 'Cultural racism in work with Asian women and girls', in S. Ahmed, J. Cheetham and J. Small (eds) *Social Work with Black Children and their Families*, London: Batsford.

Ahmad, B. (1990) *Black Perspectives in Social Work*, London: Venture Press.

Banks, S. (2004) 'The dilemmas of intervention', in J. Roche and S. Tucker (eds) *Youth in Society: Contemporary Theory, Policy and Practice* (2nd edn), London: Open University/Sage.

Banks, S. (2006) *Ethics and Values in Social Work* (3rd edn), Basingstoke: Palgrave Macmillan.

Ben-Tovim, G., Gabriel, J., Law, I. and Stredder, K. (1992) 'A political analysis of local struggles for racial equality', in P. Braham, A. Rattansi and R. Skellington (eds) *Racism and Anti-racism: Inequalities, Opportunities and Policies*, London: Open University/Sage.

Bhavnani, R., Safia Mirza, H. and Meetoo, V. (2006) *Tackling the Roots of Racism: Lessons for Success*, Bristol: Policy Press.

Bonnett, A. (2000) *White Identities: Historical and International Perspectives*, London: Prentice Hall.

Collins, P.H. (1991) *Black Feminist Thought: Knowledge, Consciousness and the Politics of Empowerment*, London: Routledge.

Davies, B. (2008) 'Reflections of youth policy: twenty-five years of *Youth and Policy*', *Youth and Policy*, 100: 5–14.

Delgado, R. and Stefanic, J. (2001) *Critical Race Theory: An Introduction*, London: New York University Press.

Ejaz, F. (1991) 'Self-determination: lessons to be learned from social work practice in India', *British Journal of Social Work*, 21: 127–142.

Garner, S. (2007) *Whiteness: An Introduction*, London: Routledge.

Garner, S. *et al.* (2009) *Sources of resentment, and perceptions of ethnic minorities among poor white people in England*: Report compiled for the National Community Forum, Communities and Local Government, www.communities.gov.uk (accessed 10 August 2009).

Gillborn, D. (2008) *Racism and Education: Coincidence or Conspiracy?*, London: Routledge.

Gilroy, P. (2004) *After Empire: Melancholia or Convivial Culture?*, Abingdon: Routledge.

Giroux, H.A. (1994) *Disturbing Pleasures*, London: Routledge.

Gunaratnam, Y. (2003) *Researching 'Race' and Ethnicity: Methods, Knowledge and Power*, London: Sage.

Hall, S. (1992) 'New ethnicities', in J. Donald and A. Rattansi (eds) *Race, Culture and Difference*, London: Open University/Sage.

Hamid, S. (2006) 'Models of Muslim youth work: between reform and empowerment', *Youth and Policy*, 92: 81–90.

Hussain, T. (2006) 'Working Islamically with young people or working with Muslim youth?', *Youth and Policy*, 92: 107–118.

Khan, M.G. (2006) 'Towards a national strategy for Muslim youth work', *Youth and Policy*, 92: 7–18.

King, E.J. (2006) 'Dysconscious racism: ideology, identity, and the miseducation of teachers', in G. Ladson-Billings and D. Gillborn (eds) *The RoutledgeFalmer Reader in Multicultural Education*, London: RoutledgeFalmer.

Kishwar, M. (1996) 'Who am I ? Living identities vs acquired ones', *Manushi*, 94: 6–17.

Ladson-Billings, G. (2001) *Crossing Over to Canaan: The Journey of New Teachers in Diverse Classrooms*, San Francisco, CA: Jossey-Bass.

Leonardo, Z. (2006) 'The souls of white folk: critical pedagogy, whiteness studies, and globalization discourse', in G. Ladson-Billings and D. Gillborn (eds) *The RoutledgeFalmer Reader in Multicultural Education*, London: RoutledgeFalmer.

Maclaren, P. (1995) *Critical Pedagogy and Predatory Culture*, London: Routledge.

Macpherson Report (1999) *The Stephen Lawrence Inquiry, Report of an Inquiry by Sir William Macpherson of Cluny*, London: HMSO, February, cm 4262-1.

Malik, R. (2006) 'British or Muslim: creating a context for dialogue', *Youth and Policy*, 92: 91–106.

Mama, A. (1995) *Race, Gender and Subjectivity*, London: Routledge.

Miles, R. (1989) *Racism*, London: Routledge.

Narayan, U. (1989) 'The project of feminist epistemology: perspectives from a non-western feminist', in A. Jaggar and S. Bordo (eds) *Gender/Body/Knowledge: Feminist Reconstructions of Being and Knowing*, New Brunswick, NJ: Rutgers University Press.

Office of Public Sector Information (2009) *The Race Relations Amendment Act 2000*, www.opsi.gov.uk/acts/acts2000/plain/ukpga_20000034_en_1 (accessed 2 October 2009).

Patel, N. (1995) 'In search of the holy grail', in R. Hugman and D. Smith (eds) *Ethical Issues in Social Work*, London: Routledge.

Patten, P. (1997) 'Racism and respect: black pride, black youth and black workers', in D. Garratt, J. Roche and S. Tucker (eds) *Changing Experiences of Youth*, London: Open University/Sage.

Sallah, M. and Howson, C. (eds) (2007) *Working with Black Young People*, Lyme Regis: Russell House Publishing.

Sivanandan, A. (2007) 'Racism, liberty and the War on Terror', *Race and Class*, 48: 45–96.

Smith, M. (1988) *Developing Youth Work: Informal Education, Mutual Aid and Popular Practice*, Milton Keynes: Open University Press.

Sue, D.W. *et al.* (2008) 'Racial microaggressions in the life experience of black Americans', *Professional Psychology: Research and Practice*, 39: 329–336.

Sue, D.W. *et al.* (2009) 'Racial microaggressions and difficult dialogues on race in the classroom', *Cultural Diversity and Ethnic Minority Psychology*, 15: 183–190.

Taylor, R., Gillborn, D. and Ladson-Billings, G. (eds) (2009) *Foundations of Critical Race Theory in Education*, London: Routledge.

Thomas, P. (2009) 'Between two stools? The government's "preventing violent extremism" agenda', *The Political Quarterly*, 80: 282–291.

Webb, M. (2001) 'Youth work with black young people', in F. Factor, V. Chauhan and J. Pitts (eds) *Working with Young People*, Lyme Regis: Russell House Publishing.

Woolett, A., Marshall, H., Nicolson, P. and Dosanjh, N. (1994) 'Asian women's ethnic identity: the impact of gender and context in the accounts of women bringing up children in east London', in K. Bhavnani and A. Phoenix (eds) *Shifting Identities and Shifting Racisms: A Feminist and Psychology Reader*, London: Sage.

Yuval-Davis, N. (1994) 'Women, ethnicity and empowerment', in K. Bhavnani and A. Phoenix (eds) *Shifting Identities, Shifting Racisms: A Feminist and Psychology Reader*, London: Sage.

Youth workers as confidants

Issues of welfare and trust

Sue Morgan and Sarah Banks

Introduction

Youth workers often form close relationships with young people who seek them out to help with personal problems. Young people discuss their feelings and actions with youth workers and expect or request that these discussions be kept confidential. Dilemmas arise when young people's wishes conflict with agency policy, other youth work values, expectations of other professionals and agencies, or when activities are illegal. Youth workers are also party to information about young people's activities that they overhear or observe during their work. Some of this information may simply be known about; some may be recorded in files. There are ethical issues around what types of information should be regarded as confidential; to whom confidentiality should be extended; what should be recorded; who should have access to records; in what circumstances information should be revealed; and whether young people should be informed.

This chapter will consider the meanings of confidentiality, how it applies in youth work in general, and in a variety of situations often encountered by youth workers including work in inter-professional and inter-agency settings. We will draw on the confidentiality literature from other welfare professions – particularly social work and counselling – where this is helpful. However, although there are many commonalities, it is important to bear in mind that the roles of youth workers are very different from those of counsellors or social workers and therefore give rise to different types of issues.

The nature of confidentiality

Confidentiality is essentially about trust. It is usually associated with entrusting someone with a secret. Since the nature of a secret is that is hidden, and few people know about it, then confidentiality is about trusting someone not to reveal this information. In the literature on professional ethics, it is often linked with the idea of privacy and the rights of those making use of professional services to determine who should have information about them, especially information they have given to professionals for a particular purpose (Clark and McGhee 2008; Cordess 2001; Tyler 2001). For example, the statement on ethical conduct in youth work published by the National Youth Agency (2004: par. 5.1.1) includes as an ethical principle that youth workers should treat young people with respect, which entails:

> explaining the nature and limits of confidentiality and recognising that confidential information clearly entrusted for one purpose should not be used for another purpose without the agreement of the young person – except where there is clear evidence of danger to the young person, worker, other persons or the community.

There are several arguments about why professional confidentiality is important in liberal societies. By 'liberal societies' we mean societies in which individual freedom is highly valued, which generally tend to be based in Western cultures located in the global North. In more collective societies, the concept of private information belonging to an individual makes much less sense and hence confidentiality between professionals and service users is not necessarily expected or respected (see Imam and Bowler (Chapter 9, this volume) for issues of cultural conflict, and Harper (2008) for an interesting discussion relating to public heath work in Nepal). Assuming a Western liberal context, Bok (1982) suggests that confidentiality can be justified with reference to four ethical principles: human autonomy regarding personal information; respect for relationships; respect for promises; and the benefit of confidentiality to society and to people needing help. As Rhodes (1986: 62–64) points out, the first three principles are interrelated and could be categorised as a Kantian justification of confidentiality – with a focus on the respect and dignity owed to each individual person. The fourth principle stresses the usefulness of confidentiality to individuals and society. If the concept and practice of confidentiality did not exist, people would not readily share information about personal and social issues and problems, and therefore might not receive the help they need (Bisman 2008: 24). If it was not possible to trust anyone to keep a secret, then the world would become a more suspicious, individualised and unfriendly place, which is a utilitarian justification based on the good social outcomes generated by confidentiality.

What is confidential information?

Often the information referred to in relation to professional confidentiality is specified as that given by service users to professionals (Shardlow 1995: 67) or 'disclosures by the patient or client to the professional' (Wilson 1978: 2). This might be interpreted as implying that confidentiality only applies to information actively given by a client, service user or participant to the professional worker. Yet this is a rather narrow interpretation of 'confidential information'. If the whole professional relationship is regarded as based on trust, then the idea of 'entrusting information' may be extended to include information that the professional gains about a service user in the course of their professional relationship, regardless of whether it is directly given to the professional. In considering what counts as confidential information in youth work, it is important to go beyond the information directly communicated by young people.

Biestek (1961: 123) gives a useful analysis of different types of confidential information in relation to social work. He defines confidential information as:

> a fact or a condition, or the knowledge thereof, pertaining to a person's private life which is normally hidden from the eyes of others.

He then divides this definition into three categories:

1   *The natural secret* is information which, if revealed, would 'defame, injure, or unjustly sadden' someone. Everyone (for example, friends, relatives, strangers or a professional) has a duty to preserve this secret. In the case of professional social and youth workers, it covers information that may have become known to a worker unofficially outside of the professional relationship.
2   *The promised secret* is where the person confided in (the confidant) gives a promise after the secret information has been revealed not to divulge it. The information may include defamatory facts as in the natural secret, or non-defamatory information of a personal nature.
3   *The entrusted secret* is information given with the previous explicit or implicit understanding that it will not be revealed. The subject matter may or may not include a natural secret and the implicit/explicit contract between the two people binds the confidant to secrecy even if the information is not defamatory. In the context of professional social work, or youth work, it is the entrusted secret that is most commonly encountered.

It seems relatively uncontroversial to regard entrusted and promised secrets as types of confidential information. Biestek's account of the natural secret, however, is more problematic. There are two ways in which a worker may come to know a natural secret. The first is in the course of professional work – for example, in a youth work setting by listening, watching or being told something by a third party. This is clearly a case where confidentiality would be expected if the information is of a 'defamatory' character. The second is outside the professional relationship – for example, at a dinner party, or when out shopping on a Saturday. Although

Biestek classifies this as 'confidential information', it may be more appropriate to regard it as 'private information' if there was no relationship of trust involved at the time the information was gained. For example, imagine a case where Jane, who has a job as a youth worker, learns during conversation at a dinner party that the father of a young woman who attends the youth club where Jane works is in prison for drug dealing. The person who revealed this information was not aware that Jane knew the young woman, and did not assume or request confidentiality. Therefore, although Jane is the recipient of sensitive information of a personal nature, it does not make sense to regard her as a confidante.

Jane may well decide it would be wrong to reveal this information to fellow workers or club members. However, this would more accurately be characterised as respecting the young woman's right to privacy, not confidentiality. This may seem merely a semantic point, but it is not. How Jane construes the nature of the information and the circumstances in which it is received may influence how she decides to use it. If Jane thinks of herself as in the role of a youth worker even when at a dinner party, and regards the information as confidential, then she may feel perfectly justified in informing her supervisor, fellow workers or recording it in a file. This is because for a youth worker employed by an agency, confidentiality usually means secret within the team or agency. By regarding it as private information, she would keep it to herself.

Applying the principle of professional confidentiality

Professional confidentiality is a complex and often misunderstood concept. In private life we often assume confidentiality to be the same as secrecy. For example, if Jane tells her friend about the details of her relationship with her partner in confidence, and the friend promises confidentiality, then Jane would expect the information to remain a secret between the two of them. In professional life matters are rarely as simple as this, since professionals often work in teams, discuss matters with supervisors and colleagues, and make recordings in shared files that are available to other professionals within and outside the agency where they work. Bond (1995: 6–7), in his research on confidentiality in multidisciplinary teams working with people with HIV, found at least four interpretations of confidentiality current among the professional staff. These ranged from absolute secrecy between the people present, through disclosure with or without permission of the person giving the information, to simply following whatever the agency or professional policy was regarding confidentiality.

Despite the much greater prevalence of multi- and interdisciplinary working in recent years and the development of numerous policies, guidelines and protocols on information sharing, differences in interpretation over what is meant by 'confidentiality' remain between practitioners in the same profession and in different professions (Ashe 2008; Baker 2008; Irvine et al. 2002). In this context, there are two important questions about how to interpret confidentiality: first, how far does the confidentiality extend; and second, when is it right not to promise confidentiality or to break confidentiality? Regarding the first question, we often talk about the worker as 'confidant' (indeed the title of this chapter uses this term), which implies that there is a one-to-one relationship between the worker and the person entrusting the information. However, this is not generally the case for professionals working in the health and welfare field where it is rare that confidentiality is confined to one person. In many cases confidentiality extends to the worker and their supervisor, or to the team to which the worker belongs, or to the whole agency, or to the agency and other professionals who work in partnership with that agency. This will depend on the practices and policies of particular agencies and workers. Even a counsellor in private practice will usually have supervision – indeed, the code of practice for professional counsellors requires this (BACP 2009).

Youth workers who are employed by an agency, whether a small voluntary agency or a large local authority, will expect to receive supervision, discuss problematic issues with colleagues and in certain circumstances (particularly suspected child sexual abuse) will be required to report serious matters to their line managers or beyond. The difference between a counsellor in private practice and an employee of an organisation is that in the case of the former the confidential information does not have to be revealed to anyone else and no action need be taken on the information received (except in very specific situations such as the prevention of terrorism, where it is legally required – see Bond 2009). The private practice counsellor is working for the client and the client should be in control of the information, respecting the core principle of client autonomy. However, in the case of workers employed by agencies, usually the worker is working to the agency's agenda as well as that of the client or service user. Part of this agenda may be about promoting the welfare of service users regardless of what they would choose themselves (e.g. preventing suicide or injury), protecting other service users (e.g. reporting an attempted theft), or serving the public interest (e.g. reporting crimes).

This leads to the second question about when it is justified not to promise confidentiality, or, if it has been promised or expected, when to break it. If we pay attention to cases when we should not promise confidentiality, then there may be fewer situations arising when confidentiality has to be broken. For example, the Code of Ethics of the British Association of Social Workers BASW (2002: par. 4.1.7 (d)) states that confidential information should only be revealed with the consent of the service user,

> except where there is clear evidence of serious risk to the service user, worker, other persons or the community, or in other circumstances judged exceptional on the basis of professional consideration and consultation, limiting any such breach of confidence to the needs of the situation at the time.

The National Youth Agency (2004: par. 5.1.1) suggests that confidentiality should be respected except in situations where 'there is clear evidence of danger to the young person, worker, other persons or the community'.

The possibility of danger or harm and the concept of 'working in the public interest' are the clauses that generally override the commitment to confidentiality. These give workers permission either not to offer confidentiality, or to break it in specific cases. If an agency has a clear policy on when confidentiality cannot be assured, this makes it easier for workers. Agencies may also have policies about the types of information that workers have a duty to reveal. Nevertheless, it is sometimes hard to decide what makes a situation dangerous enough to warrant the divulging of personal information. Workers may face dilemmas in deciding whether to prioritise the principle of respecting young people's rights to make their own choices or to divulge confidential information against young people's wishes in the interests of promoting their own or others' welfare or challenging oppressive practices.

While confidentiality is important in maintaining trust and respecting individual rights to self-determination and privacy, youth workers and other welfare professionals also regard it as important that underlying inequalities and oppressive practices are exposed and tackled in local communities. This may entail prioritising other ethical principles or concerns above the maintenance of confidentiality – for example, preventing abusers from exploiting young people; openly discussing and addressing issues of drug dealing; and recognising and preventing bullying, violence and harassment. As the report of the National Policy Round Table (2008) in England on gang, gun and knife crime states: 'Approaches must involve young people and their communities in shaping an understanding of problems and agendas for positive action.' Similarly, in cases of sexual violence, as Churchill and Honning (1997: 66) argue: 'safety and sexual violence is a community issue, it's everyone's responsibility and the community can support victims by acknowledging the issues and providing support.' In the case of youth work, practitioners have conversations with young people that develop learning about how structural inequality impacts upon their personal lives. They want to enable young people to understand that their difficulties, while experienced at an individual and personal level, are often rooted in broader political and social issues.

Young people's understanding of confidentiality

We will now consider some of the specific features of youth workers' roles that may differentiate them from other welfare professionals. Characterised as informal educators (see Chapter 1), most youth workers do not tend to have formal one-to-one encounters with individual young people in the way that social workers and counsellors do, unless they are working in specific youth counselling, advice or other projects involving casework. So there is less chance to explain the nature of confidentiality to young people, or to establish a 'contract' setting out expectations. Since youth workers work informally and often in a relaxed way, they may not be perceived by the young people as 'professionals' and young people are less likely to understand how youth workers are accountable to their employing agencies. They may be perceived more as 'friends' than as professional workers. There may be misunderstanding about the nature of the role, relationship and the extent of confidentiality. A youth worker's manner is likely to be friendly, open, encouraging and respectful, and some young people may not be used to meeting professionals who treat them like this. It may easily be assumed that everything revealed is secret to the people present.

Revealing information picked up during the work: issues of drugs and alcohol

Young people often behave very differently with each other than when they are with their parents/carers. Youth workers witness such behaviour, with an understanding that the details of this behaviour (unless it is dangerous) are confidential within the youth work project. Frequently in youth work settings young people talk about drugs and alcohol. Youth workers are likely to understand young people's drug use in a context of their disillusionment, low expectations and inequality. They will understand young people's attempts to achieve 'adult' status, which seems to be conferred through drinking and taking drugs. Conversations between youth workers and young people about drugs and drinking are commonplace. Young people often want to talk privately about their levels of consumption and behaviour while under the influence. Young people will only have these kinds of conversations if they are confident that the worker is not going to report them to the police, their parents/carers or schools.

However, there are situations when it is impossible for youth workers to keep information about drugs confidential – for example, if they become concerned for the immediate safety of young people and judge them incapable of making sound decisions. If someone is in danger, having taken too much or having a bad reaction, a youth worker will usually consider their plea for confidentiality far less important than the need to prevent injury or save their lives, and so inform parents/carers and/or arrange for them to be taken to hospital. If the danger is more long term, and if the young person has consistently failed to seek help, then workers may consider it their duty to inform parents/carers. The age of the young person is significant and would affect workers' judgements about their responsibility to the parents/carers. Youth workers would approach parents/carers with the expectation that they would be concerned and supportive, but it may be wrong to assume this.

The duty to keep confidences is balanced by considerations for the safety of others. Workers may hear who the drug dealers in a local community are.

Difficulties in keeping this confidential may arise if the dealer is known to be unscrupulous – for example, mixing drugs with more dangerous substances, dealing to children, or being involved in acts of violence to procure drugs or pay for them. Reporting dealers whom the wider community may perceive as providing a useful service to them could make it difficult for workers to maintain relationships or even their presence in this community. It may make them inaccessible to the very people whose needs they could most usefully serve.

The following example (Case study 10.1) was recounted by a youth worker who had been working informally with a group of young people who were taking drugs. This is a case where the worker had information that he had picked up in the course of his work (a natural secret).

Case study 10.1

A youth worker employed to work in a youth centre in an inner city area had been conducting some detached work with a group of about twenty young people aged 14–20 years old who congregated on street corners near the centre. They had a passion for rave music, and over half of the group admitted to using drugs. The group complained of boredom, so a contract was drawn up with them enabling them to use a room in the centre twice a week to play their music. They agreed that no illegal substances would be brought into the centre and that they would not come in under the influence of drugs. With the odd exception this agreement was kept, and the worker began working with a subgroup on issues around drugs. Problems emerged when a drug dealer known to some of the young people started hanging around outside the centre. Due to his close contacts with the young people, the worker had information that would be likely to lead to the arrest of the dealer. Colleagues and the majority of the members of the centre's management committee urged the worker to go to the police. The worker knew that this would mean losing contact with the young people and being labelled as a 'grass'. He felt he had been making some headway with them on harm reduction strategies.

This case involves conflict between a worker's view about what he should do (maintaining the trust of a small group of individuals), and the views of others in his agency (catching a drug dealer in the broader public interest). While the fact of the dealer hanging around was public knowledge (the management committee members knew about this) it was the details of his activities known by the worker which would determine whether he was caught by the police or not. What the worker eventually did might not only depend on how strongly he stuck to his principle of confidentiality, but also whether he thought the police would actually catch the dealer and how much good that would do in terms of reducing drug use in the area compared with the harm that would be done to the productive work he was doing with this group of young people (utilitarian considerations).

This example is framed as an ethical dilemma for the youth worker: he has to make a difficult ethical choice between two courses of action – should he inform the police or not? While ultimately the choice is his, it is not a decision he has to take alone. The worker's supervisor or manager should also help to consider the possible consequences of any course of action and offer support. There may be a good relationship with a community police officer who could deal with the situation tactfully. Joint work with local drug and alcohol projects could help identify options. In an ideal world, it would be good practice to involve the young people in deciding what to do – enabling them to take some responsibility for the situation and working through the possible options themselves. Talking to the young people about the dilemma, and developing a relationship of openness, honesty and respect would be part of the informal educational process of youth work; yet it might also put the worker at risk of reprisals from the dealer. This example demonstrates the multitude of issues that lie behind what seems to be a simple choice about whether or not to reveal a natural secret.

Revealing information to prevent harm: issues of crime and violence

The kind of confidential information youth workers regard as most serious and provoking most anguish is that relating to cases where young people are involved in activities that might cause them, or other people, serious harm and/or which is against the law or public interest. Youth workers mention self-harm, drug use, crime, under-age sex and sexual and physical abuse. The dilemmas raised in these situations usually relate to balancing young people's rights – to privacy; to freedom to determine their own actions; to have their confidence respected (derived from Kantian principles) – against the rights or interests of particular others or society as a whole (utilitarian considerations). Rhodes (1986: 64) argues that the principle of 'protecting society' may often outweigh individuals' rights to autonomy and privacy. However, the breaking of a confidence is regarded as serious because it usually involves a betrayal of trust, or at least the potential loss of trust of the young people being worked with.

Often youth workers work in communities where low incomes and poverty are the norm. Education about how inequality operates in society is a crucial area of work for youth workers, and the discussions in which they involve young people have important implications. They will seek to make the relationship between crime and inequality explicit and relevant. While youth workers are increasingly expected to provide 'positive activities' to divert young people from crime, it is the active and conscious choice to refrain from criminal activity that is the youth work aim. Workers and young people are acutely aware of the pressure brought to bear by consumerism and the marketing of products and promotion of ideals which most people cannot afford or achieve. Many young people feel that their standing within their peer group depends on wearing expensive designer clothes, having a new mobile phone, the latest music and games equipment. Advertising both creates and feeds on young people's sense of inadequacy, and youth workers have a responsibility to enable young people to understand how this happens and how it affects them.

Youth workers may find young people offering them stolen goods and the services of shoplifters. It is not only wrong for youth workers to be involved in theft but it would undermine the work they do on issues of equality. Youth workers need to demonstrate to the people they work with, not that they are morally superior, but that their dialogue on the issue is not influenced by their own self-interest. As Jeffs and Smith (2005: 96) argue, this is the 'moral authority' from which flows the right of youth workers to be listened to. Youth workers also serve as role models for young people so they need to strive to ensure that their own behaviour matches that which they advocate. Workers must be alert to the possibility that by keeping illegal or morally wrong activities confidential, they may inadvertently convey that these activities are acceptable, as illustrated by Case study 1.1. It is important to see confidentiality in the wider context of the youth work role. This involves developing young people's trust in the worker not just as someone who will not 'grass', but as someone whose opinions can be respected and who can engage in conversations exploring difficult issues.

Youth workers may become aware of many different kinds of activities that might be classified as illegal or criminal taking place within local communities such as: people working while claiming benefits, under-age sex, carrying knives, shoplifting, under-age drinking, domestic and other violence, dealing in stolen goods or drug dealing. If youth workers reported to the police all the crime that they hear about, their presence in communities would not be tolerated. A worker would be likely to report criminal activity to the police in situations when safety is threatened.

Case study 10.2

In the youth club one evening, a youth worker saw a 15-year-old male member looking at something shiny and then placing it in his rucksack. The young man did not see the worker, who wondered if the shiny object was a knife. The club had a policy that no weapons were allowed in the club and anyone bringing one in would be reported to the police. The youth worker had a good relationship with the young man and felt he could safely approach him to talk. When asked, the young man affirmed that he had a knife in his bag and said that he had taken it from his younger brother earlier to stop him getting into trouble. He asked the youth worker not to tell his parents or the police and offered to hand over the knife.

This is not a case of a young person spontaneously volunteering personal information to the youth worker; it is a case of the youth worker finding out, through his own observations, about a young person clearly breaking a club policy, and the young person then requesting that this be kept secret. In a situation like this, how a youth worker responds will vary according to the assessment of immediate danger; the young person's mood and behaviour; and the workers' relationship with the young person. Quite likely a youth worker in this situation would have a conversation with the brother, then with both boys and then with their parents/carers. Judgements would be required about the credibility of information, when intervention is necessary and what is appropriate. The worker would probably discuss this with the youth work team as the situation developed. Knowledge within the youth work team of the circumstances of the brothers would influence what that intervention might be. They might discuss how the policy applies in this case and consider if reporting to the police and parents was appropriate. Each situation is different and a blanket approach may not always be useful. Youth workers understand the very negative consequences of young people getting a criminal record and often want to help them avoid this. Yet, if the club has a policy, it will be important to respect this. Parents/carers of the young people attending the club may know about the policy and feel reassured that no weapons are allowed, and that if their children are caught with weapons they will be told. If the youth worker does not carry out the policy and someone is subsequently injured, this would be a very negative outcome. If the young man had given the knife to the youth worker it would be negligent to return it to him. If the worker feels the policy is inadequate, then he should bring this to the attention of the agency managers in order to improve it, make it relevant and provide further guidance about how to handle such situations. Work on the issue of knife crime would probably be prioritised for the project.

Revealing information to prevent harm: issues of abuse, self-harm and suicide

Where young people are in danger, youth workers' responses are guided directly by their employers as part of safeguarding and child protection procedures. All local authorities and most voluntary agencies in Britain have very clear policies requiring workers to report any cases of young people at risk of serious harm. Yet such policies can seem inadequate in practice when responding to a very upset young person talking about their problems.

Ethical problems and dilemmas may arise for youth workers in cases where a young person is unaware of the workers' inability to keep certain types of confidences – for example, relating to information about potential abuse. If the young person had known that the worker would report the information given, he may not have told the worker. Regulations often warn youth workers against promising confidentiality. This can present a difficult decision relating to the point in the conversation when the worker tells the young person that he cannot keep the confidence. Workers may be afraid of a very adverse reaction from the young person. Some may not tell them at all, waiting until after the young person has gone before informing their safeguarding 'lead officer' or their manager. This can be criticised as irresponsible, making the situation easier for the worker by avoiding a difficult conversation, and giving the young person no choice in how the situation is approached. A worker following this line of action also loses the chance to inform the young person of the way the procedures work and what will happen. It contradicts the youth work commitment to respecting and empowering young people.

The Code of Ethics developed in New Zealand by the National Youth Workers' Network Aotearoa (2008) seeks to avoid this situation. This Code states:

> The young person's ability to trust the Youth Worker to hold information in confidence is fundamental to the relationship. When it is clear that confidences might be shared, the Youth Worker will explain the boundaries of confidentiality. These boundaries will take into account the requirements of their organisation, the young person's culture and the setting Youth Work is carried out in (such as rural and specific cultural communities).

This Code attempts to ensure that young people understand what will happen as a result of what they tell and aims for a position where workers will only receive informed disclosures from young people. This statement recognises the dynamic that culture brings to understanding. Paying attention to the cultural context is important, as it seeks to avoid assumptions and ensure young people's full comprehension of all the implications. This practice gives young people choice about what they reveal and hopefully a larger say in determining their own future. However, it does imply that young people may choose not to disclose. In such circumstances the youth worker must be vigilant to direct them to other sources of support and monitor the situation closely to avoid continuing abuse and suffering.

Uncertainty can cloud the issues of abuse and self-harm, and there is often fear of repercussions for an inappropriate response. Workers may worry that if a young person is lying about abuse, they too may be accused. Accusations of abuse, even when unsubstantiated, have the power to wreck youth workers' lives and careers (Nicholls 1995:163).

Many experienced youth workers doubt the effectiveness of the safeguarding procedures. No matter what youth workers judge to have happened, they are not entitled to diagnose abuse: even if they report an actual disclosure, this is regarded only as suspected abuse. Young people frequently withdraw disclosures made to youth workers when faced with the more formal structures of the police and local authority children's services and a fuller understanding of the consequences of their assertions, and how this will impact upon their different family members and home life. In such cases it could be difficult for them to return to the youth project and so this source of support can be lost.

Equally difficult ethical dilemmas and problems arise when young people tell youth workers they are engaging in risky or self-harming behaviours, or even that they may be thinking about suicide. The following example (Case study 10.3) was given by a female youth worker.

Case study 10.3

While clearing up after an evening youth work session, a 15-year-old young woman, Dawn, approached the youth worker and asked if she could have a word in private. Dawn said she couldn't go on any longer. She hated her life. She showed the youth worker scars on her arms and told the youth worker how she cut herself. She pleaded with the worker not to tell anyone. The worker later reflected:

I felt apprehensive and unsure. I felt as though I could make this situation much worse by saying or doing the wrong thing. Although I understood our policy about reporting such serious concerns, and had taken training in self-harm, these did not help me when faced with this young woman in distress. I knew I had to tell my manager, but I felt this would start a process that would put this young woman under even more pressure before she could receive any relief. It might make things worse before they could get better. I felt as though what I said and did could determine whether or not she made it through the night.

The worker's comments suggest that she sensed the importance of the moment for the actions of the young person. She was keenly aware that simply following the policy (reporting the disclosure) did not guarantee a constructive response or good outcome. She felt a strong sense of responsibility for the well-being of the young person. She thought that the wrong response might influence the young person to act on her suicidal feelings.

The main issue identified in this example by the worker is not whether to report the young woman's suicidal thoughts – the worker knows she will tell others and find help for the young woman. The issue is what kind of conversation to have next and whether, when and how to tell the young woman that the worker will have to take some action. This is a practical question about what is the most effective approach to take to ensure the young woman's welfare. It requires moral qualities in the worker of professional wisdom, courage, sensitivity and empathy.

Ensuring that the agency policies and procedures are followed adds another dimension of stress into an already intolerable situation. The worker will be mindful of various sources of relevant advice, such as: 'sometimes it is necessary to go against a child or young person's expressed wishes in their best interests' (DfES 2005: 9). Yet she also knows that this consideration must be balanced against the possibility of making the situation worse. The government information-sharing guidance states: 'inform the person that the information has been shared . . . if it would not create or increase the risk of harm' (DCSF 2008: 7).

In cases involving suicidal feelings, a situation can quickly deteriorate, as Gutierrez (2006: 130) comments:

> Suicide risk is a fluid construct, affected by many factors which may change dramatically from moment to moment, making accurate assessment a significant challenge and prediction of future behavior a near impossibility.

This is a very heavy burden for a youth worker to shoulder, and as Tyler (2001: 82) points out, in such cases: 'No worker should have that responsibility without at least discussing this suicidal person and their role anonymously with someone else.'

Hill (1995) urges workers who are in contact with young people to talk about such issues rather than be afraid that such talk will provoke them into action. Youth work with young people who self-harm identifies that the issue of control is very important (Green 2001; Kirk 2007; Smalley et al. 2004). Mindful of this, and of the urgency of the situation, what the youth worker in this example actually did was to ask the young woman to meet her the following day. She reassured her that she would try to help her to find ways to improve her life. She discussed the service of the Samaritans (a helpline) and gave her their telephone number. The project had leaflets about self-harm and details of a support group and, by giving these to the young woman, the worker was able to convey a sense of understanding and hope. She helped the young woman to identify a friend whom she could text or call through the night if she needed to.

When a young person has disclosed information about a potentially dangerous situation a youth worker will usually seek to share this immediately with a colleague or supervisor, so that they can check that their response is appropriate and effective.

In a stressful situation it is easy to make mistakes. It is important that workers develop an understanding of the dynamics of their own reactions and motives when they feel that a young person needs their help. Mander (1997: 35) writes of counsellors: 'the image of the good shepherd associates easily with the Pied Piper, the false prophet, the charismatic fanatic.' Sanders (1996: 43) argues that the harmful side of the motive to help can be the desire for dependency. The helping relationship must not be distorted to meet the needs of the helper.

Working with other professionals and agencies

In many countries multi-agency and multi-professional approaches to working with young people are increasingly being adopted. Such approaches are a particular feature of policies for children and young people in England, with the development of inter-professional working through 'integrated' services, where professionals from different agencies work closely together. In this context, for example, the needs of individual children and young people may be assessed by a range of professionals (including youth workers) using a common assessment framework, which enables information to be stored and shared among agencies, with the young people's or parents'/carers' consent (Children's Workforce Development Council 2009: 59–63). A national database is also being developed, designed to record basic identifying and contact details of all children and young people and showing which agencies are working with them. Although 'explicit, informed consent of the child or young person (or parent/carer if acting on their behalf) will be required to record contact details for a sensitive service' (Department for Children, Schools and Families 2009: 2), these developments raise very challenging issues for youth workers. What information can be shared and what must be kept confidential to youth workers and/or to their employing agencies? Who has access to the electronic records being compiled?

Joint protocol agreements about information sharing between partners help to clarify roles and make explicit to young people what information sharing involves. For example, agencies working with homeless 16- and 17-year-olds in County Durham developed a joint protocol for information sharing and published a leaflet for young people (County Durham Joint Protocol 2009). The development of inter-professional working brings with it the need for clear definitions of roles and boundaries, as youth workers and youth work agencies now routinely work with police officers, social workers, health workers, teachers and their employing agencies. How can youth work aims and principles be understood and respected by other professionals and other agencies? Are all professionals and all agencies equal partners in the relationships? Case study 10.4 illustrates some of these points.

Case study 10.4

Two youth workers based in a school but with an area remit had been working on a detached youth work project in a seaside village. The project was a response to political pressure 'to do something' about a large group of young people who gathered on the beach in the evenings. The young people generally behaved well. Although there were a few instances of drinking, mostly the young people just wanted to be together, in a large group, as they were accustomed to do at school. Youth workers established good relationships with the group members, whom they felt were in danger of becoming unreasonably criminalised. A minor incident with one young man drinking led to images of members of the group being captured on surveillance cameras. Youth workers were asked to meet with police and school leaders, shown video footage of the group and asked to identify the young people. They felt they received little understanding of or respect for their role as youth workers from the other agencies.

Some youth workers feel that one consequence of the move to inter-professional and integrated working is that one of youth work's core values – to strive for positive change and equality within society – is unrecognised if not altogether lost. Case study 10.4 shows how partner agencies and professionals expect youth workers to act as agents of control. Prior work with partners, outlining youth work's aims and principles, may have helped avoid this misunderstanding. Discussion about each partner's expectations of the others is very important. It is important that youth workers have confidence in their values and clarity about the role and purpose of youth work. This is necessary to enable them to refuse inappropriate requests for information and to avoid being co-opted into control functions that jeopardise the values and distinctiveness of youth workers' roles as informal educators (see Banks (2009) for an example of the dilemmas faced by a youth worker in a youth offending team).

Many youth workers are concerned about the increasing amount of information being compiled and stored about young people. As Hoyle (2008) comments:

The concern with 'joined-up services', monitoring the behaviours of children and young people, and the sharing of information has led both to the construction of databases that are often unknown to them, contain intimate material on a scale that has been deemed disproportionate by the Information Commissioner; and to the ability of a wide range of people to access that information. In addition, it has drawn a range of practitioners (including many informal educators) into the formal surveillance process. There has been a fundamental cost to this. Children and young people are being denied spaces to explore feelings, experiences and worries away from the gaze of the state.

It is important that youth workers and their managers think seriously about what records should be kept and why; and when and to whom records or files should be shown.

Conclusion: developing ethical practice

Skills in handling confidentiality are increasingly recognised and required as core competencies for youth workers in many countries (see Lifelong Learning UK 2008; New York City 2008). Yet each situation is different and calls for thought and careful judgement. Thorough knowledge of policy and procedure is required but the application of this is unlikely to be routine or comfortable. Rarely are there easy solutions, and decisions often need to be revisited and reworked. Youth workers striving to maintain their integrity and ongoing conversations with young people about consent will increase the likelihood that the youth work relationship remains intact and useful throughout the process. Focusing on the possibility of violating confidentiality highlights key areas of planning. Consideration of circumstances that might arise will result in advance preparations, which can have a beneficial impact in a crisis situation. The following suggestions may be useful for those working with young people.

Working with young people

- Fostering dialogue about confidentiality with young people will inform their expectations of workers.
- Having useful resources available such as leaflets about issues like self-harm and suicide will help allay young people's sense of isolation and workers' sense of powerlessness.
- Work with young people to help them identify and consolidate their support networks reduces the level of dependency on the relationship with the youth worker.

- Promoting the work of agencies that can keep confidences directs young people to places where they can have confidential discussions while trying to decide on a considered course of action (for example, in Britain this includes Childline and the Samaritans. International organisations can be identified through *befrienders.org*).

Working within the youth work team

- Teams of youth workers can plan how to work together to support a colleague having a 'private' conversation with a young person.
- It is important to ensure that the availability of advice and support for youth work staff at the times when they are working with young people is embedded in the structure of provision.
- Induction for new workers and ongoing training for all staff should establish and update understanding of procedures and identify sources of support. Everyone should have a working knowledge of policy and procedures about safeguarding and confidentiality, which should be reviewed regularly. Adequate supervision to enable reflection and learning should be available to all youth work staff.
- Workers could usefully consider possible scenarios and reflect upon actual experience from a broad range of perspectives: that of the young person, their friends, parents/carers, teachers, police, youth work managers and colleagues, the youth work organisation, and others with interests in the situation. They should consider how their words, actions and judgements might be perceived by others.
- It is vital to consider the contexts of diversity and culture, and how these might impact upon situations and shape understanding and practice.

Working beyond the team

- It is important to communicate the principles, values and ways of working of youth workers, youth work agencies and projects to other professionals and agencies working with the same young people.
- Building relationships with child protection staff and other agencies at a local level informs workers' understanding of how scenarios may unfold.

Questions for reflection and discussion

1 In what circumstances might it be ethically justified to break confidentiality when working with young people?

2 Imagine yourself in the shoes of the youth worker(s) in one of the case studies in this chapter. What ethical issues would the situation raise for you? What actions would you take and how would you justify these ethically? What resources would the youth workers need (such as conversational skills and team support) in order to decide what to do and then implement their actions?

3 What are the advantages and disadvantages of close working relationships between different professionals working with young people? How can respect for young people's freedom of choice and privacy be maintained in the context of increasing sharing of information, as illustrated in Case study 10.4, when the police asked youth workers to identify young people?

Recommended reading

Bok, S. (1982) *Secrets. On the Ethics of Concealment and Revelation*, New York: Pantheon. This is a classic text written by a philosopher on the concept of secrecy.

Clark, C. and McGhee, J. (eds) (2008) *Private and Confidential? Handling Personal Information in the Social and Health Services*, Bristol: Policy Press. This is an edited collection with useful chapters on confidentiality and privacy in the welfare professions, including a chapter by Ashe on working with children and young people.

References

Ashe, P. (2008) 'Working with children and young people: privacy and identity', in C. Clark and J. McGhee (eds) *Private and Confidential: Handling Personal Information in the Social and Health Services*, Bristol, Policy Press.

Baker, C. (2008) 'Working together? Sharing personal information in health and social care services', in C. Clark and J. McGhee (eds) *Private and Confidential: Handling Personal Information in the Social and Health Services*, Bristol, Policy Press.

Banks, S. (2009) 'Values and ethics in work with young people', in J. Hine and J. Wood (eds) *Work with Young People: Developments in Theory, Policy and Practice*, London: Sage.

Biestek, F. (1961) *The Casework Relationship*, London: Allen & Unwin.

Bisman, C. (2008) 'Personal information and the professional relationship: issues of trust, privacy and welfare', in C. Clark and J. McGhee (eds) *Private and Confidential: Handling Personal Information in the Social and Health Services*, Bristol: Policy Press.

Bok, S. (1982) *Secrets. On the Ethics of Concealment and Revelation*, New York: Pantheon.

Bond, T. (2009) *Standards and Ethics for Counselling in Action*, 3rd edn, London: Sage.

Bond, T. (1995) *Confidentiality about HIV in Multidisciplinary Teams*, Newcastle: Northern and Yorkshire Regional Health Authority.

British Association of Social Workers (BASW) (2002) *The Code of Ethics for Social Work*, Birmingham: BASW.

British Association for Counselling and Psychotherapy (BACP) (2009) *Ethical Framework for Good Practice in Counselling and Psychotherapy*, Lutterworth, Leicestershire: BACP.

Childrens' Workforce Development Council (2009) *The Common Assessment Framework for Children and Young People: A Guide for Practitioners*, Leeds: Childrens' Workforce Development Council, www.dcsf.gov.uk/everychildmatters/strategy/deliveringservices1/caf/cafframework (accessed July 2009).

Churchill, H. and Honning, T. (1997) 'Student safety matters',*Youth and Policy*, 56: 64–68.

Clark, C. and McGhee, J. (2008) *Private and Confidential? Handling Personal Information in the Social and Health Services*, Bristol: Policy Press.

Cordess, C. (ed.) (2001) *Confidentiality and Mental Health*, London: Jessica Kingsley.

County Durham Joint Protocol for Homeless 16 & 17 year olds (2009) *Sharing Information About You*, Durham, UK. guide for practitioners

Department for Children, Schools and Families and Communities and Local Government (2008) *Information Sharing: Pocket Guide*, www.dcsf.gov.uk/everychildmatters/resources-and-practice/IG00340/ (accessed July 2009).

Department for Children, Schools and Families (2009) *ContactPoint Q&A*, www.dcsf.gov.uk/everychildmatters/strategy/deliveringservices1/contactpoint/about/contactpointabout/ (accessed July, 2009).

Department for Education and Skills (DfES) (2005) *Effective Communication with Children, Young People and Families*, www.dcsf.gov.uk/everychildmatters/strategy/deliveringservices1/commoncore/effectivecommunicationengagement/communication (accessed July 2009).

Green, K. (2001) 'Finding your own voice: social action groupwork with young people who are suicidal and self harming', *Youth and Policy*, 71: 59–76.

Gutierrez, P. (2006) 'Integratively assessing risk and protective factors for adolescent suicide', *Suicide and Life-Threatening Behavior*, 36 (2):129–135.

Harper, I. (2008) 'Confidentiality in practice: non-Western perspectives on privacy', in C. Clark and J. McGhee (eds) *Private and Confidential: Handling Personal Information in the Social and Health Services*, Bristol: Policy Press.

Hill, K. (1995) *The Long Sleep*, London: Virago.

Hoyle, D. (2008) 'Problematizing Every Child Matters', *The Encyclopaedia of Informal Education*, www.infed.org/socialwork/every_child_matters_a_critique.html (accessed May 2009).

Irvine, R., Kerridge, I., McPhee, J. and Freeman, S. (2002) 'Interprofessionalism and ethics: consensus or clash of cultures', *Journal of Interprofessional Care*, 16: 199–210.

Jeffs, T. and Smith, M. (2005) *Informal Education*, 3rd edn, Derby: Education Now Books.

Kirk, E. (2007) 'Edges and ledges: young people and informal support at 42nd street', in H. Spandler and S. Warner (eds) *Beyond Fear and Control. Working with Young People who Self Harm*, Ross on Wye: PCCS Books.

Lifelong Learning UK (2008) *National Occupational Standards for Youth Work*, www.lluk.org (accessed September 2009).

Mander, G. (1997) 'Towards the millennium: the counselling boom', *Counselling*, February: 32–35.

National Policy Round Table (2008) *Report on Gang, Gun and Knife Crime: Seeking Solutions*, www.nya.org.uk/shared_asp_files/ (accessed March 2009).

National Youth Agency (2004) *Ethical Conduct in Youth Work: A Statement of Values and Principles from the National Youth Agency*, Leicester: The National Youth Agency.

National Youth Workers' Network Aotearoa Inc. (2008) *Code of Ethics for Youth Work in Aotearoa New Zealand*, Wellington,NYWNA, www.youthworkers.net. nz/CoE0book.pdf (accessed July 2009).

New York City Department of Youth and Community Development (2008) *Core Competencies for Youth Work Professionals*, www.nyc.gov/html/dycd/downloads/pdf/core_competencies_for_yw_professionals.pdf (accessed October 2009).

Nicholls, D. (1995) *Employment Practice and Policies in Youth and Community Work*, Dorset: Russell House Publishing.

Rhodes, M. (1986) *Ethical Dilemmas in Social Work Practice*, Boston, MA: Routledge & Kegan Paul.

Sanders, P. (1996) *First Steps in Counselling*, Manchester: PCCS Books.

Shardlow, S. (1995) 'Confidentiality, accountability and the boundaries of client–worker relationships', in R. Hugman and D. Smith (eds) *Ethical Issues in Social Work*, London: Routledge.

Smalley, N., Scourfield, J., Greenland, K. and Prior, L. (2004) 'Services for suicidal young people', *Youth and Policy*, 83:1–17.

Tyler, M. (2001) 'Developing professional practice', in L. Richardson and M. Wolfe, *Principles and Practice of Informal Education*. London: Routledge.

Wilson, S. (1978) *Confidentiality in Social Work, Issues and Principles*, London: Free Press.

<table>
<tr><td>11</td></tr>
</table>

Youth workers as researchers

Ethical issues in practitioner and participatory research

Janet Batsleer

Introduction

This chapter will explore the range of ethical dilemmas confronting youth workers who engage in practitioner and participatory research. In this context, 'practitioner research' refers to research conducted by practising professionals with 'insider knowledge' of the subject they are studying. 'Participatory research' refers to research that involves people who might traditionally have been 'studied' and seen as 'research subjects' acting as researchers themselves, alongside a principal practitioner and/or academic researcher.

Research undertaken within a participatory and critical framework is unlikely to be chiefly concerned with the production of 'social facts'. The truths it is likely to disclose are usually inter-subjective and derive from the attempt to produce shared meanings and shared understandings. Whether youth workers initiate the research, or act as 'gatekeepers' to enable others to negotiate access to community groups and young people, or work as partners or co-researchers with stakeholders, they will need to clarify their own roles and the issues of power, participation and voice that are posed by the research project.

This chapter will move from a discussion of the parallels between the roles of youth workers as informal educators and as practitioner researchers to investigate the current debates about the role of 'evidence' and 'knowledge' in youth work. It will explore some of the critical issues routinely faced by practitioner researchers engaged in a negotiation of power: issues of control of agendas, of informed consent, of partnership working, of authority in the interpretation of data, of the recognition of complexity and of support to marginalised voices and perspectives. It will become clear how far the dilemmas of practitioner research mirror the dilemmas of informal education practice.

Ethics of practitioner research in informal education

Participatory enquiries are closely aligned with methodologies which have been commonly used in youth and community work. However, in common with all participation, participatory collaborative enquiries exist along a continuum of involvement. By virtue of their professional role, it is unlikely that youth workers would support research that did not embrace some form of dialogue with young people. However, the forms of engagement with young people in research are varied and may include youth workers playing a role in:

- offering simple facilitation to enable young people to undertake their own research; this may include training in research methods;
- supporting young people to work alongside adults as researchers in various forms of community audit;
- enabling adult researchers to gain access to young people, including facilitating critical dialogue with a young people's reference group;
- engaging with young people as part of a research project through in-depth interviewing using open questions;
- entering into dialogue with young people about the findings of significant periods of time spent in participant observation and listening.

The more informal educators see themselves as committed to unsettling the every-day and taken-for-granted forms of knowledge of a group, the more the question 'and why do you think that?' will form part of their dialogues. Involvement in research projects will then be a clear development from existing youth work practice.

There are parallels at every point between the practice of informal education and the practice of research. The skills of asking questions in research enquiry build on the skills of listening and engagement that youth workers use. The period of analysis with which any period of youth work engagement begins is mirrored by the question of 'in whose interests?' a body of research is being undertaken. The use of group work as a basis for learning through association is a good basis for the development of participatory, collaborative enquiry. The voluntary rela-tionship that is the starting point for informal learning is mirrored in the 'informed consent' necessary for any research process. The need for trustworthiness in the practitioner is echoed in the commitment to honesty and reliability in research. The importance of sensitivity in research touches on the role of accompaniment, guidance and support in youth work. Finally, practitioners' commitments to empowerment and to young people's coming to voice demand attention to adult/ young person power dynamics and to responsibility in the representation of commonality and difference in the reporting of research findings, especially in relation to minority and marginalised perspectives. So, in asking about the ethical dilemmas facing youth workers as researchers, this chapter assumes a competence in negotiating ethical dilemmas already present in professionals with a bent towards curiosity and enquiry in relation to young people.

Knowledge: for social improvement or social control?

Researching – that is, enquiring, asking questions and developing systematic new knowledge and understanding about a social issue, an area or a group of people – has been part of the practice of community and youth work from the beginning. University Settlement members and the staff of the late Victorian Charity Organisation Society could be described as some of the early social scientists of modern urban life (Gilchrist *et al.* 2003). By the mid-twentieth century, the study of sociology and the study of youth were linked through a preoccupation with the presence of 'gangs' in 'street corner society' and a desire to document and understand the lives of young people who posed a challenge to the mainstream of society (Whyte 1943). In the late 1960s and early 1970s detached youth work projects were closely linked with the 'radical criminology' of the National Deviancy Symposium (Taylor and Taylor 1972). Voluntary youth organisations such as the Youth Development Trust in Manchester set up projects to research and highlight need which was invisible to policy-makers (YDT 1970). 'Knowing' has long been linked to the desire for social change. Researchers have been seen as allies in developing agendas for the benefit of young people and have been made welcome.

However, researching and 'intelligence gathering' about neighbourhoods and particular groups of young people has also been seen as threatening. Providing intelligence on young people's deviant or criminal behaviour did not necessarily lead to improvements in life chances but might give the forces of the law a not altogether welcome access to particular neighbourhoods. Once social scientists were linked through public policy initiatives to psychological or public health researchers in uncovering 'indicators' for a whole range of pathologies such as 'juvenile delinquency', drug abuse, teenage pregnancy, alcohol consumption and worklessness, asking questions and researching was as likely to become 'labelling' as 'empowering'. It could and does also lead to a sense of particular neighbourhoods and issues being 'researched to death'. 'Knowing' has been linked to control, containment and measurement or simply irrelevant time wasting in ways that mean researchers are sometimes regarded not as allies but as a nuisance, unwelcome or more actively as a threat.

Who knows?

In the early twenty-first century dilemmas of research need to be understood in the context of the 'knowledge explosion' and the 'knowledge economy'. The generation of knowledge about young people and about the social world they inhabit is now critical to making money through advertising and marketing. This model of knowledge through focus groups has been adopted by service providers engaged in commissioning and developing services in the 'efficient' market-based models of service delivery. It sometimes seems as if questionnaires, scales and indicators of satisfaction accompany every transaction and every moment in practice. The capacity to store postcode-based information through computer technology makes it possible for my 'taste' in consumption to be calibrated with terrifying accuracy. 'Knowing' is part of good business. This kind of 'knowing' may also be used to predict the life chances and, crucially, determine the expectations set for children and young people in particular neighbourhoods. Perversely, indicators set as a result of calibration of deprivation may lead to a systematic lowering of expectations for young people in the poorest neighbourhoods.

Accompanying this explosion of knowledge within the economy, there has been an intensification of the roles of researchers, an expansion of the university sector and of the range of sources of funding for research. Charitable foundations – such as the Joseph Rowntree Foundation in Britain – with their roots in the model of social enquiry to support progressive social change still exist. Research councils continue to fund independent research led by senior academics, and professional associations of academic researchers publish ethical guidelines and standards for research. Ethical guidelines are a vital safeguard because so much research is now commissioned by government or public bodies with very clear 'vested interests', often in achieving an evidence base, through evaluation, for an already established policy direction to which resources have been allocated. 'Knowing' becomes part of a process of policy-making and part of the struggle for resources within the state. It may be argued that the definition of 'evidence' adopted by public bodies in commissioning services enables the health sector to be the chief beneficiary from the investment of public funds for social purposes; research models for measuring, testing and evaluating the impact of services are well established there. 'Knowing' is part of policy-making and resource allocation.

Finally, a further transformation in the conditions of 'enquiring' and 'knowing' is represented by the development first of the television and now of the internet as sources of popular knowledge. Examples include the use of the narratives of popular soap operas to convey public knowledge; the status of celebrities who advocate 'knowledge' (to the people); the facilities of Google and other internet search engines that enable us to ask and find answers to any question but without any apparent way of checking with the 'authorities' what is reliable knowledge and why. All these give a dizzying context to the contemporary efforts of youth and community workers to build on the tradition of enquiry and 'knowing' as part of their practice. In fact, honesty and reliability in the attribution of sources of knowledge is a fundamental ethical requirement of research without which the development of knowledge ceases to be a reliable and trustworthy process. It is for this reason that plagiarism is regarded with such horror as a fundamental breach of ethics throughout the academic world. At the same time, the academic conventions of peer review (as the source of authority) in contributions to learned journals, encyclopaedias and dictionaries are under pressure from more apparently democratic spaces for the construction of knowledge such as *Wikipedia*. 'Knowing' is everywhere and is as popular as the pub quiz. So research and 'knowing' seem neither welcome nor unwelcome but simply ubiquitous and hard to discern.

Changing definitions of 'youth'

At the same time as the change in conditions of research and 'knowing' there is a concomitant transformation in understandings of childhood and youth. Until recently children and young people were understood as 'objects' of research who should be treated with consideration and respect but whose involvement with research was largely on the basis of adult and parental agreement and consent, if any consent was thought necessary. It is now generally recognised that young people can be active subjects and participants within the research process. In what Nick Lee (2005) calls 'the new paradigm' children and young people are not seen as 'human becomings', but as 'human beings'. Put simply, what this means is that young people's perspectives form part of the research process throughout and are taken seriously as a form of knowledge. The recognition of 'situated knowledges' (Haraway 1988; Harding 1992) enables practitioner researchers to locate the sources of knowledge they are developing without recourse to positivism on the one hand or highly contestable accounts of 'false consciousness' on the other. It enables attention to be paid to issues of power, plurality, oppositional voices and multi-vocality accompanied by a recognition of the complexity of 'truth' in the social domain. It is no longer straightforwardly the case that the 'adult' authority interprets and makes sense of young people's lives on behalf of young people. Young people are part of a dialogue with adult researchers. Adult and 'expert' authority does not disappear, but the specific situated knowledges which young people bring to the research process are recognised (Jones 2004).

This is the large context in which the ethical foundations and dilemmas of research in youth and community work need to be discussed. Yet the research that youth and community workers undertake will usually be small-scale and limited in scope. The student dissertation or community audit (Packham 2008) may be the first occasion on which a youth and community worker engages with research. However, the contexts in which youth workers will find themselves undertaking research on their own behalf or contributing to larger-scale research projects include playing roles as 'gatekeepers' to communities that others may wish to investigate and as co-instigators of research led by young people or community groups. The ethical issues in research explored in the rest of this chapter will make reference to each of these contexts.

Conflicting interests?

Two of the most important questions for a practitioner researcher are: 'Who is the research or enquiry designed to benefit?' and 'Whose agendas are being served by it?' In the case of small-scale research such as that usually undertaken for a Bachelors or Masters degree, it is likely to be primarily the interests of the researcher that are served by the research, both in the narrow sense of enabling them to achieve a personal goal of accreditation and in the wider sense of being led by a commitment to independent enquiry on a subject of personal choice. Research undertaken as part of studies of this kind is generally regarded as offering 'training' in research methods rather than as liable to produce reliable and trust-worthy knowledge. So it is not usually subject to scrutiny by research committees, although the proposals are generally approved by academic supervisors, and students may have to complete research ethics forms designed to minimise harm to participants and researchers.

In the case of invitations to participate in larger-scale funded research, it is likely that the sponsors of the research already have an agenda and it is a matter for ethical investigation to determine whose interests are being served by this agenda. Who needs to know what and why? And how does this sit with the commitment of youth and community work practice to a young person-centred agenda? It is also likely that the researchers will develop their proposals in relation to pro-fessional guidelines. In Britain, this may include ethical guidance published by the British Psychological Society (BPS 2006), British Sociological Association (BSA 2002), British Educational Research Association (BERA 2004) or the Social Research Association (SRA 2003). Research proposals will be subject to scrutiny by research ethics committees (or institutional review boards) of the health service, local authorities, other agencies or the higher education institution to which the researchers are affiliated.

Cases of conflicts of interest in the framing of research and enquiry are wide-spread, as the following example shows. The need for the national government in Britain to gather information and intelligence about terrorist networks has led to approaches to youth work agencies to become involved in research and intelligence gathering in relation to a strong current political agenda connected to 'combating violent extremism'. Youth work as a discipline is highly subject to political agendas and, like many political agendas and perhaps more than most, this one seems to be a self-evident good. It also seems to be the case that the current intelligence-gathering strategies being used by government authorities are less than satisfactory. Youth workers already live and work 'under the radar' or in the places where 'deep dives' for intelligence gathering are deemed to be needed. However, the intensification of the stereotyping of Muslim communities and therefore the increasing alienation of young people and adults from 'mainstream' services and opportunities seems to be a direct consequence of such agendas. In consequence, youth work managers need to decide whether involvement with such research would lead to their alienation from Muslim communities, whose members might be labelled as potential terrorists. The ethical reasoning undertaken requires active discussion and dialogue with young people as stakeholders from a range of communities, in particular with young Muslims who might be damaged as a result of the intensification of stereotyping. Where a decision to go ahead has been taken, it has been in the belief that this offered a significant means of empowering young people to challenge the terms of the debate. This proved to be the case in work undertaken by the North West Regional Youth Work Unit in England with a young people's reference group leading a project that investigated the impact of stereotyping on communities.

Deciding which research to become involved with draws on the same approach to ethical dilemmas as the youth worker might face in other aspects of practice, demanding careful consideration of which decision will best support the commitment to social justice and flourishing and to the enabling of informed choices which underpin both youth work and community development (Packham 2008). Youth workers may be called on to equip young people with research skills such as questionnaire design or the planning of focus groups while the same young people are denied access to discussion of the larger contexts for research and evaluation. In this context, moral reasoning about the nature of the research process and young people's own role as stakeholders with perspectives on the issue in hand will become part of the decision-making about involvement.

Young people's involvement in research is not just about a series of techniques but inevitably requires young people's participation in ethical and political reasoning. Conflicting agendas may not only derive from national and international policy contexts, or from the agendas of particular pressure groups, charities or campaigns; they are also likely to be generated locally. They may result from conflicts among older and younger people in a locality or among competing community projects and groups. The whole issue of antisocial behaviour, young people's groups or 'gangs' and their activities is a complex area of negotiation. Neighbourhood 'community clean-up' campaigns of a variety of types may involve research into 'positive activities' or diversionary strategies for young people who are by no means misbehaving. Youth workers have often made strategic and ethical decisions, preferring to dedicate their research time to supporting young people seeking to limit the use of 'mosquitoes' (the teen alarms designed to prevent young people from gathering in public spaces) and other dispersal devices, and have decided to act not just on a local but a national basis.

Engagement with young people from the beginning in creating baseline accounts and identifying research questions or suggesting different (either complementary or contradictory) lines of enquiry mitigates against the effect of agendas that are led by powerful stakeholders, whether this is in a student dissertation or a funded research project. The importance of developing good questions cannot be understated and enabling good questions to be asked is a fundamental skill of critical education. However, the participation of young people in agenda-setting does not of itself address the ethical questions of 'in whose interests?' research is being under-taken as the power of powerful discourses in part resides in their ability to become part of the everyday common sense of their times. What 'everybody knows' or 'everybody thinks' needs to be treated with caution and the question 'in whose interests' needs to be addressed, whatever the source of the research agenda.

Research that leads to flourishing

Following the Nuremberg Code (1947), the principles of doing no harm through research, always linked to principles of voluntary informed consent and the right to withdraw from research processes, are central to all research codes of ethics. For example, the Statement of Ethical Practice of the British Sociological Association (2002: pars 11 and 13) includes the following guidance:

> Although sociologists, like other researchers are committed to the advance-ment of knowledge, that goal does not, of itself, provide an entitlement to override the rights of others.

> Sociologists have a responsibility to ensure that the physical, social and psychological well-being of research participants is not adversely affected by the research.

Ethical debate about the practice of informal education is itself concerned with the *ends* of informal education. Some practitioners and theorists emphasise the goal of enabling a young person's ability to choose, while others emphasise that informal education is a process of social education that aims to support a young people's flourishing. The practitioner researcher in informal education therefore needs to be clear whether they will remain content with a negative definition of 'no harm' in relation to young people's well-being, or whether they seek more positively to contribute to young people's flourishing. It is also possible that areas of harm through research may exist even when there is an overt intention to promote flourishing. This has been discussed particularly in relation to 'harm-minimisation' approaches to risk in work with young people. For example, researchers may be concerned to understand young people's risky behaviour in cases of self-harm, eating disorders or binge drinking. Therefore they may convene a group of young people to discuss coping strategies, which may prompt a renewed interest in or engagement with the risky behaviour among the young people (Spandler and Warner 2007). Furthermore, while researchers cannot take respon-sibility for the use to which their research results may be put, they can certainly be expected to consider the possible effects of the dissemination of their research results in making decisions about enquiry and in informing participants of possible harmful effects. In relation to research on sensitive subjects, including research involving matters generally regarded as personal and private and/or disclosure of criminal activity, there is a particular need for researchers to be aware of their responsibility to young people's well-being. Where material is discussed which may cause distress it is important to create an alliance between practitioners and researchers so that the young person is not left without support (Renzetti and Lee 1993).

Informed consent

The principle of voluntary informed consent is a key feature of ethical practice in social research. According to the British Sociological Association (2002: pars 16 and 17):

> Voluntary informed consent implies a responsibility on the sociologist to explain in appropriate detail, and in terms meaningful to participants, what the research is about, who is undertaking and financing it, why it is being undertaken, and how it is to be disseminated and used.

> Research participants should be made aware of their right to refuse participation whenever and for whatever reason they wish.

The principle of voluntary informed consent makes sense to informal educators whose own practice is developed through voluntary relationships with young people. However, the use of 'carrots' to encourage young people to take part in a project and to achieve consent needs consideration. If giving sweets or cigarettes to young people as part of a process of engagement is unacceptable, how acceptable are the gifts of cash or vouchers for high street shops which may replace such incentives? At what point do gifts to participants in a research process compromise the knowledge gained in such an enquiry? It is widely recognised that payment of expenses for inconvenience and time lost is not designed to be an inducement, and it is on this basis that expenses are paid to research participants. However, this needs case-by-case discussion. In research with young people (generally understood as those aged 14 to 19) it is increasingly recognised that they are able to consent to involvement in research in their own right, without need for further consent from parents. However, the ability of a young person to give free and uncoerced consent to taking part in a research process is subject to the constraints of power relationships which frame the work, even when young people are being encouraged to be active participants in shaping the research agenda, analysing data and disseminating the results of research.

In the case of research with young people with learning disabilities, or experiencing stressful life or health problems, it may be that their ability to understand what is being asked of them in terms of their participation in a research project will mean that the researcher needs to gain consent from the parents, guardians or carers.

However, the idea that informed consent and anonymisation alone can mitigate against the abuse of the power relationships which are implicit in research and knowledge production is a fantasy. It is to the ethical responsibility of the practitioner researcher to address the power dynamics and the situatedness of their research process that we now turn. In a world in which there is also a great deal of emphasis on personal control of and access to personal information stored in electronic forms, there are ethical issues concerning the safe storage of data and its anonymisation when used in publication. Yet anonymity may not be the preferred strategy of some research participants, who may value the opportunity to give voice, in their own words and in their own names, to the knowledge which is of such value to the researcher. It all depends on the analysis of power and how it is being handled in the research process.

Power, inclusivity and marginality

In the development of youth and community work practice there is a long history of commitment to a practice of informal education which is empowering and inclusive, and which challenges marginalisation and oppression. Practitioners have been prepared to take steps to ally themselves and their work with the experiences of the most marginalised participants. In doing this, they may be thought to be giving up any claims to be able to act rigorously, impartially and reliably as researchers. They seem to commit the grossest of errors in terms of current models of knowledge: they already know the answers; they have jumped to conclusions; they have taken sides. It is in order to address this 'problem of knowledge' that a number of contemporary feminist philosophers have developed what has become known as 'standpoint epistemology' (Harding 1992). This involves making explicit the power of the researcher's own position (their situatedness) and taking responsibility for the decisions which they make in constructing representations of the world. It also involves an active commitment to dialogue with many positions different from one's own. Practitioner research projects require dialogue with a range of stakeholders who will form reference groups for research projects. The dialogue in these cases will be multi-faceted and arise from a commitment to partnership. In the case of research with young people, it means an active commitment to dialogue between the adult researchers and the not-yet adult participants in the research process. It requires recognition of the different meanings associated with different starting points.

This places a responsibility on researchers to identify or create safe environments within which to undertake research with young people (including ensuring that all researchers have standard criminal record checks). They need to work at expressing the purposes and goals as well as the processes of the investigation in ways that the young people with whom they are working can understand. Furthermore, the power dynamics between adults and young people can create a sense of 'obligation to participate'. This needs to be carefully monitored if 'participation' is not to become a form of coercion. Dialogue about and communication of research findings also need to be undertaken in a respectful manner even when the findings may appear to be less than flattering or less than advantageous to the research participants. There needs to be clarity about the responsibilities and authority claims of researchers in representing their findings.

In the processes of recruitment of research participants, particularly in small-scale research, there needs to be an acknowledgement of the limitations of the researchers' own networks. 'Young people' are not a homogeneous group. The social divisions, exclusions and patterns of marginality which occur throughout societies are also present among young people, in specific historical forms. Sometimes there is a need to emphasise the significance of minority voices and to allow the research process to amplify and validate perspectives which are not often heard in the mainstream. This means deliberately seeking out the perspectives of young people who do not form a majority in the group being engaged with and valuing those voices by recognising them as potential sources of knowledge. This validation of the 'coming to voice' of frequently ignored peoples is a major preoccupation of critical social research and yet it needs to avoid becoming a 'giving voice': that is, a coercive 'putting words into people's mouths'.

Another important aspect of such research is the 'denaturalising' or 'denormalising' of taken-for-granted power relationships and revealing the historical specificity and situatedness of forms and relationships which may seem to 'have always been this way'. This might include young person-directed research into adult norms; women researching masculinity; or black scholars depicting 'whiteness'. These are examples of ways in which critical researchers have been able to 'turn the tables' of knowledge and power. In representing the results of the research and its findings, it is therefore valuable to express how young people and adult researchers have been involved in the interpretation of data so that their relative contribution to the research process can be discerned and evaluated by readers.

Conclusion: Who needs to know? What can she know?

Critical enquiry into matters which affect young people and their communities will continue to form an important part of the practice of informal educators. They will also need to continue to engage with work conducted by expert researchers about young people, research which will be conducted for a range of purposes. In particular, practitioner researchers will be required to act as gatekeepers of young people's involvement in evaluation and monitoring (which can themselves be seen as forms of research) as 'young people's participation' becomes a requirement of the funding of commissioned services. The more that various public bodies set out to induce young people to 'take part', the more the spaces for research agendas generated elsewhere than in the policy centres are closed down. Yet knowing is so closely linked to power that a simple rejection of involvement in these public agendas must surely be linked to the generation of alternative agendas drawn from much more extended dialogue with young people.

The alliance between adults and young people and the forms this alliance can take in the development of research projects is critical to their success. The operation of power means that the experience of challenging research agendas is usually a profoundly unsettling one. It is far less unsettling to find ways of encouraging young people to participate in existing agendas than to engage in that process of challenge. When a particular perspective has been silenced for a long time, bringing that perspective to voice can feel dangerous, and the clash between mainstream perspectives and those that are emerging through research can lead to a period of 'feeling crazy' in which nothing seems to make sense. This has been documented in particular by feminist researchers and in the context of critical race theory (Delgado and Stefganic 2001; hooks 1997; Lather 1991). All researchers – young or old – need support in working through these moments, and as in youth work, so in youth work-based practitioner research, the process of accompaniment is critical.

Since young people are unlikely to be accepted as experts in the generation of reliable and trustworthy knowledge (they have not undertaken sufficient training; their education is not sufficiently developed), the role of the adult advocate on behalf of young people's ways of knowing also remains important. The way in which the adult researcher represents and interprets the findings which have been generated through their conversations with young people may be understood as a form of advocacy. The philosopher Lorraine Code (1991) has argued that in current conditions of inequality, the role of the advocate continues to be more powerful than self-advocacy by subordinated groups, as the knowledge of the less powerful is continually treated as suspect and lacking credibility by the guardians of expertise. Thus the role of advocate is required to strengthen the credibility of less powerful voices. The skilled practitioner researcher working alongside young researchers in a supportive and advocacy role strengthens rather than undermines young people's coming to voice and dialogue. The youth worker as researcher will continue for some time to come to also be the youth worker as advocate.

Questions for reflection and discussion

1   Why do honesty and trustworthiness matter in practitioner research and how can they be established?

2   What resources and processes are needed to enable practitioners and researchers to ask good questions?

3   What are the tensions for youth workers in seeing practitioner research as a form of advocacy?

Recommended reading

Fraser, S., Lewis,V., Ding, S., Kellett, M. and Robinson, C. (2004) *Doing Research with Children and Young People,* London and New Delhi: Sage. This book includes a wide range of current discussion of issues in research. Many chapters, including a useful chapter by Priscilla Alderson, discuss ethics.

Layard, R. and Dunn, J. (2009) *A Good Childhood. Searching for Values in a Competitive Age,* London: Penguin. This major study by The Children's Society incorporated reference groups of young people in each of its research themes and is worth considering as an example of research as advocacy.

Percy Smith, B. and Thomas, N. (eds) (2009) *A Handbook of Children and Young People's Participation: Perspectives from Theory and Practice,* London: Routledge. This book engages in thought-provoking ways with strategies for representing young people's voices in a direct way in research reporting.

References

British Educational Research Association (BERA) (2004) *Ethical Guidelines*, www.bera.ac.uk/blog/category/publications/guidelines/ (accessed July 2009).

British Psychological Society (BPS) (2006) *A Code of Conduct for Psychologists*, www.bps.org.uk/the-society/code-of-conduct (accessed July 2009).

British Sociological Association (BSA) (2002) *Statement of Ethical Practice*, www.britsoc.co.uk/equality/Statement+Ethical+Practice.htm (accessed July 2009).

Code, L. (1991) *What Can She Know? Feminist Theory and the Construction of Knowledge,* Ithaca, NY: Cornell University Press.

Delgado, R. and Stefganic, J. (2001) *Critical Race Theory: An Introduction*, New York: New York University Press.

Gilchrist, R., Jeffs,T. and Spence, J. (eds) (2003) *Architects of Change: Studies in the History of Community and Youth Work,* Leicester: The National Youth Agency.

Haraway, D. (1988) 'Situated knowledges: the science question in feminism as a site of discourse on the privilege of partial perspective', *Feminist Studies,* 14: 575–599.

Harding, S. (1992) *Whose Science? Whose Knowledge? Thinking from Women's Lives,* Ithaca, NY: Cornell University Press.

hooks, b. (1997) 'Representing whiteness in the black imagination', in R. Frankenberg (ed.) *Displacing Whiteness,* Durham, NC: Duke University Press.

Jones, A. (2004) 'Involving children and young people as researchers', in S. Fraser *et al.* (eds) *Doing Research with Children and Young People,* London: Sage.

Lather, P. (1991) *Getting Smart. Feminist Research and Pedagogy With/In the Postmodern*, New York: Routledge.

Lee, N. (2005) *Childhood and Human Value,* Buckingham: Open University Press.

Nuremberg Code (1947) reprinted online, www.hhs.gov/ohrp/references/nurcode.htm (accessed July 2009).

Packham, C. (2008) *Active Citizenship and Community Learning*, Exeter: Learning Matters.

Renzetti, C.M. and Lee, R.M. (eds) (1993) *Researching* Sensitive *Topics,* London: Sage.

Social Research Association (SRA) (2003) *Social Research Association Ethical Guidelines*, www.the-sra.org.uk/ethical.htm (accessed July 2009).

Spandler, H. and Warner, S. (2007) *Beyond Fear and Control: Working with Young People and who Self-harm. A 42nd Street Reader,* Ross on Wye: PCCS Books.

Taylor, I. and Taylor, L. (eds) (1972) *Politics and Deviance: Papers from the National Deviancy Conference*, Harmondsworth: Penguin.

Whyte, W.F. (1943) *Street Corner Society: Social Structures of an Italian Slum*, Chicago, IL: University of Chicago Press.

Youth Development Trust (YDT) (1970) *Young and Sick in Mind,* Manchester: YDT.

<table>
| 12 |
</table>

Young people as activists

Ethical issues in promoting and supporting active citizenship

Jason Wood

Introduction

Over the past decade there has been increasing policy attention in many contemporary liberal democracies to developing young people as active citizens. Schools and informal educators provide programmes of citizenship education, and youth workers are increasingly charged with implementing projects that strengthen young people's political, social and moral engagement with local, national and global issues.

The ideas of active citizenship are very familiar to youth workers. One of the long-standing cornerstones of practice has been to 'empower' young people through active participation. Much of this work draws on a rights-based approach to working with young people. However, the promotion of young people's active citizenship is often imbued with contradictions. On the one hand, there are calls for the greater participation of young people and on the other, there is a tendency to frame young people as lacking the capacity to exercise these responsibilities.

This chapter briefly defines how citizenship is understood in contemporary policy and practice, and examines how youth workers promote active citizenship. In doing so, it considers some of the ethical issues practitioners face in these attempts, focusing particular attention on questions of purpose and strengthening young people's voices. The chapter concludes with questions that are designed to stimulate further critical reflection.

What is active citizenship?

It is not the intention of this chapter to explore the origins and development of citizenship, nor to examine in detail the policy context of active citizenship education. However, for the purposes of setting this chapter in context, a brief overview of some important concepts is offered here.

Citizenship is a complex concept and one that is contested and difficult to define. It has no essential or 'universally true meaning' (Crick 2000: 1). In its current usage it concerns 'membership', usually attached to a state. It is also a normative ideal (Coffey 2004), a 'set of practices . . . which define a person as a competent member of society' (Turner 1993: 2) with qualifying, associated rights and responsibilities. It concerns a *status*:

> Bestowed on those who are full members of a community. All who possess the status are equal with respect to the rights and duties with which the status is endowed.
>
> (Marshall 1950: 28–29)

A basic definition of citizenship therefore entails an understanding of three interrelated aspects: the *status* of citizenship and what this status ensures by way of the *rights* and *responsibilities* that belong to those who hold it. Each of these three components is explored in turn.

The *status* of the citizenship concerns who is regarded as a citizen and of what they are members. In most modern definitions there is recognition that we can hold citizenship of different communities at different levels. As local citizens, we are members of our immediate neighbourhoods, towns and cities. At a national level, we are members of a nation state which is responsible for determining and upholding our rights and responsibilities. For those living inside the European Union, we are further governed and hold membership at a supranational level as European citizens. Finally, in an era of increased globalisation, it is almost a common phrase that we are all global citizens now. These multiple layers of citizenship ensure that defining citizenship remains complex and sometimes contradictory as we exercise rights and responsibilities at the different levels.

The second aspect of citizenship concerns the *rights* that are guaranteed to the person holding the status of citizen. The modern rights debate often focuses on the extension of universal social and civil rights. An equally powerful debate in UK social policy and one that is specific to young people is the extension of rights to 'be consulted', 'have a say' and 'be involved' (Children and Young People's Unit 2001; Fleming and Hudson 2009; Hine 2009). The opportunities and capacity of young people to be consulted about and to shape public institutions are often framed as rights, and these stem from Article 12 of the UN Convention on the Rights of the Child 1989 (of which the UK is a signatory) which states:

> State parties shall ensure to the child who is capable of forming his or her own views the right to express those views freely in all matters affecting the child, the views of the child being given due weight in accordance with the age and maturity of the child.
>
> (UNICEF 2008)

Finally, there are the *responsibilities*, duties or obligations that citizens must fulfil as part of their status. Responsibility is a vast concept that can take many different forms. It may include the duties we have at a neighbourhood level to act with social and moral responsibility to others. We have a responsibility to work and pay taxes, and these responsibilities are often linked to our right to access welfare. Our responsibilities as global citizens also take on increasing importance. For example, global warming, now almost universally accepted as a real consequence of industrialisation, represents a significant risk to sustainable life. Yet, by far the biggest response by governments is not found in the scaling back of industrial development. It is in the education of its citizens to make more prudential choices about their energy use and household waste disposal.

The entitlement to rights and the discharge of responsibilities, particularly in respect of political and work obligations, suggest an *active* component to citizenship. Crick (2000: 2) argues that active citizenship is a focus on both the 'rights to be exercised as well as agreed responsibilities'. Active citizens are people who are:

> Willing, able and equipped to have an influence in public life and with the critical capacities to weigh evidence before speaking and acting.
>
> (Crick 2000: 2)

Increasingly, young people demonstrate 'activity' through volunteering, engagement with public services and democratic participation (Andrews *et al.* 2008; Crick 2000; Heater 2004; Lister 2003) and, in the context of this chapter, active citizenship concerns the qualities, behaviours, attitudes, values and activities that are expected of young people in order to fulfil expectations of membership.

Promoting young people's active citizenship: the context

The promotion of young people's active citizenship has become a key policy concern in many advanced liberal democracies. This concern has often been informed by evidence arguing that young people are lacking certain attributes expected of active citizens. Two particular policy issues are often argued to be responsible for the drive towards promoting young people's active citizenship: these are young people's political engagement and the perceived problem of antisocial behaviour (Wood 2009a). Each are now discussed in turn.

A feature of contemporary democracy is a preoccupation with the disconnection between citizens and the political processes designed to govern them. It is argued that there is an entrenched 'democratic deficit' (Jeffs 2005) that suggests democracy is 'in crisis' (Coleman 2006). Young people's political participation in particular attracts much political and academic debate. Claims are made that 'young people are estranged from conventional politics and are becoming increasingly politically apathetic' (Wallace 2003: 243). Voting behaviour is often cited as an indicator of political engagement and, across Western and Northern Europe, young people aged between 18 and 29 are generally the least likely to vote (International Institute for Democracy and Electoral Assistance 1999). Wider still, there is evidence of a growing youth disengagement in 'new and old democracies alike' based on global turnout statistics (Ballington 2002).

The detachment of young people from the formal democratic processes invites competing claims for the cause of this phenomenon. Some commentators argue that there is an entrenched apathy within the age group (Wilkinson and Mulgan 1995) with claims that young people care only about themselves (Pirie and Worcester 2000). Other explanations include alienation (Roker *et al.* 1999), a decline in trust (Mulgan and Wilkinson 1997), and cynicism and scepticism (Wring *et al.* 1998).

However, there is much counter-evidence to suggest that young people are engaged in a range of alternative forms of politics through issue-led campaigns, such as environmental activism or movements to promote social justice. As a result, many participate in politics through demonstrations, signing petitions or joining international campaign groups. Across Europe, for instance, there is evidence of young people's involvement in political activism, especially in resistance movements or challenges to government rule (Wallace 2003). For Furlong and Cartmel (2007), this is not a new development since young people throughout history have often displayed different forms of civic engagement. As a consequence, Wallace (2003: 244) argues that 'we may be looking at the wrong things when prematurely announcing the disengagement of young people from politics'. None the less, since voting behaviour is the dominant measure of political engagement, the declining rates of participation among young people are the most frequently used indicators that stimulate a policy response.

The issue of political engagement is supplemented by a concern with young people's moral and social behaviour. In the UK context, this has led to a pre-occupation with addressing antisocial behaviour through increased civil and criminal measures (see Yates 2009). While young people have long been subjects of adult anxiety (France 2007), at no other time in history has their behaviour been so regulated (Wood 2009a). There is an increasing focus on the 'pre-criminal': aspects of young people's social and moral behaviour that may be classified as antisocial. New laws are designed not to *address* criminal activity but to *prevent* it through measures located at the site of the individual and the community. Moreover, this drift concerns itself with incivility: behaviours that were once distasteful are reframed as antisocial, and potentially criminal. Often these measures are targeted at young people who 'hang around' in their local neighbourhoods and estates. In surveys that measure the perceptions and experience of antisocial behaviour, young people 'hanging around' is often cited as the biggest concerns for adult participants (see e.g. Upson 2006). Yet, as readers will be aware, for young people the process of 'hanging around' is often undoubtedly *pro*-social. Being part of a local community and friendship group is important for a young person's identity development, and research suggests that young people exhibit a strong attachment to the local neighbourhood (Weller 2007).

Taking both problems together, we begin to understand the motivations behind different strategies that seek to engage young people as active citizens. On the one hand, the problem of democratic disengagement is countered by efforts to teach young people about politics both in the classroom and through experience-based learning. On the other hand, young people are increasingly encouraged to take an active part in their neighbourhoods in order to demonstrate socially responsible membership of the community.

The impression then is that the policy drivers for young people's participation are often based on a deficit model of young people which labels them as lacking qualities that need to be addressed by practitioners. However, those in the business of youth work may take a different view. As Roberts (2009: 53) notes, 'taking part is central to youth work' and there has been a long-standing commitment to participative work.

Youth work has historically been understood as an educative process concerned with facilitating young people's development as active citizens. In real terms, this has often been interpreted as entailing process models where practitioners work with young people to increase the 'level' of involvement they have in, say, the running of a local youth club. Huskins (2003) visualised this as a 'curriculum development model' where young people progress through seven stages of empowerment, from the limited end of 'making contact' through to 'leading'. Another common way of illustrating youth work participation is in the form of a 'ladder' where participation is progressed through 'steps' towards greater autonomy (Simpkin 2004). Such approaches can be criticised for their tendency to see participation in simplistic and linear terms, and critically the 'danger of creating some sense of failure if the high rung on the ladder is not reached' (Simpkin 2004: 15). None the less, they offer evidence that youth workers seriously consider the relationship between participation and empowerment.

In his review of how youth work promotes active citizenship, Rowe (1999: 58) found that most practitioners did not relate to the term 'citizenship' since it tended to imply for them 'passive conformity to the status quo'. However, many practitioners engaged regularly in forms of rights-based education and were in favour of strategies that sought to emphasise responsibilities to self and others as 'vital to the achievement of a tolerant and humane society' (Rowe 1999: 59).

Having briefly established that young people's active citizenship is of concern to policy-makers, and that youth workers have long committed themselves to promoting young people's effective engagement, we turn now to two important questions that practitioners need to consider in their efforts.

Asking 'why?'

The question at the heart of all social policy interventions and one that frequently concerns reflective youth workers is: *why* am I engaging in this work? Associated questions include *what* do I want to achieve as a result of my interventions in a young person's life, and ultimately *who* benefits? In the process of ethical dialogue, we consider the reasons why we engage and this often involves balancing our own personal values with those of our profession, alongside the drivers that shape and prioritise our work (such as national policy or organisational objectives). Sometimes these can be competing perspectives on our role: 'tensions' that we learn to manage (Tyler 2009).

This tension is apparent in citizenship education. We have already established that youth workers have a commitment to promoting participation by empowering young people to take a more active role in their own lives and the worlds they occupy. However, many youth workers will claim that they do more that just stimulate an active role. According to the National Occupational Standards for Youth Work, practitioners encourage and enable young people to 'influence the environment in which they live' (Lifelong Learning UK 2008, value 10). Youth workers go beyond mere awareness raising to support effective political change (Wood 2009b). By fostering environments where critical thinking and action can flourish, practitioners support young people to 'claim their right to influence the society in which they live' (Young 1999: 22).

However, even a cursory review of the policy context of citizenship education reveals something of a different message in terms of how we understand government motivations. The dominant message here appears to be one of young people 'failing' to live up to expected standards, both in their political and their social engagement. Where examples of activism occur, they are sometimes deemed to be unacceptable or problematic by adults, and this further cements the idea that young people are irresponsible.

There are some examples we can draw upon to illustrate how such tensions might manifest in practice.

Case study 12.1

A group of young people wanted to challenge the closure of the local community centre. The local centre housed a voluntary youth club which young people in the area had been attending. The club was staffed by a youth worker who was paid by the local authority to work with the young people. However, due to a city services reorganisation, the centre was to close and the club relocated to a centre in another neighbourhood.

Young people expressed concern that the club would now be over two miles away and in an area where they would not normally go.

The closure of the community centre offered a valuable opportunity for the practitioner to support young people in a form of political education and activism: a credible example of meaningful participation work. In supporting the young people to challenge the closure, this could build young people's skills and awareness of activism, and also provide a realistic insight into the possibilities and problems of democracy insofar as the young people may not be successful in their campaign (Wood 2009b). However, this work might not be judged in the same way by the local authority that simultaneously paid the practitioner to work with young people *and* was responsible for the closure. The ethical dilemma for the practitioner came with determining which side of the fence to sit on: whether to actively support the young people in their campaign or to support the young people in dealing with the closure.

Case study 12.2

When citizenship education was first instituted in the UK during 2002 and 2003, the consequential increase in debate about social issues in schools was widely reported as a beneficial and welcome development. However, when in the same year schoolchildren staged a series of 'school strikes' to attend anti-war protests against Britain's involvement in the Iraq War, this action was condemned by many teachers and their concerns were amplified in the media. Children and young people participated in 'what were, for most, their first political demonstrations' (Brooks 2003: 41). Yet the dominant view of the educational establishment was that 'the strikes represented an "unruly" excuse to truant' (Cunningham and Lavalette 2004: 259). Headteachers wrote to parents to assure them that schools were not sanctioning protests (BBC 2003a) and in some cases, students were formally disciplined through suspension (BBC 2003b). One headteacher from a school where some 60 pupils staged a walk-out reflected a common response to the protests in calling them 'irresponsible and dangerous . . . whoever organised this across the schools was fantastically irresponsible' (cited in BBC 2003a).

Claims of young people's irresponsibility were debunked by several interviews conducted by researchers and journalists at the time. There was evidence in abundance of coherent arguments put forward by young people to justify their involvement in the demonstrations that was reflective of goals of citizenship education: namely, a concern for international issues, the importance of human rights and a 'concern for the common good' (Advisory Group on Citizenship 1998: 44). Thus,

> In a country where children and young people are thought to display high levels of political apathy, the justifications that pupils gave for their actions were remarkably considered, reasoned and articulate; indeed, they almost precisely reflected the key values and dispositions that . . . form the core of citizenship teaching.
>
> (Cunningham and Lavalette 2004: 260)

This second example illustrates that young people had decided to take action about an issue of particular importance to them, and that this had ultimately clashed with their attendance at school. Cunningham and Lavalette found that young people identified such action as *responsible* in the face of being seen as *irresponsible* by teachers. The educational establishment had argued that the less contentious evidence of higher levels of debate in the classroom was evidence in itself of responsible citizenship.

It is hard to argue that both the response to the community centre closure and the school strikes were anything less than a sign of exemplary active citizenship on the part of young people. Many youth workers might applaud such activity as indicative of effective political education and meaningful participation, and can offer similar examples. However, this depends on what is determined to be the *purpose* of citizenship education. Is it to promote and foster the conditions of democratic behaviour, even where this may challenge structures and institutions such as the youth worker's paymasters? If not, then what is citizenship education for?

Whereas the tradition of citizenship education and participation is closely aligned to the need for greater political involvement, in recent times and certainly in the UK context, for many, citizenship education has become another strand of education for moral and social responsibility. The model of citizenship education used in English schools, for instance, identifies strongly with a civic republican tradition of citizenship with its emphasis on political duty and responsibility (Annette 2008), though it goes somewhat beyond political participation. The aims of citizenship education include strengthening 'social and moral responsibility', suggesting an interest in the development of good character. On this model, assessing good character and morally responsible young people is largely evidenced through their respect for authority and for others, as opposed to their ability to think critically and challenge established norms, as discussed by Young (Chapter 6, this volume).

Thus, on the one hand, the purpose of citizenship education might be the development of young people's political literacy and their capacity to understand, influence and challenge the processes of decision-making. On the other, it is seen as an instrument for strengthening socially and morally responsible behaviour. Where this becomes problematic is if we accept the dominant deficit model of young people which implies that they are somehow 'outside' of social and moral norms. These twin purposes have the potential then for confusion and contradiction. As Davies (2001: 307) notes, citizenship education seeks:

> On the one hand, to foster compliance, obedience, a socialisation into social norms and citizen duties; and on the other, to encourage autonomy, critical thinking and the citizen challenge to social injustice.

This apparent contradiction is found throughout youth policy. As Williamson (2009: 139) notes, UK policy:

> Swings from conceptualising young people as valued citizens, through suggesting a sense of their vulnerability, to perceiving them as villains. Simultaneously it promotes their participation and demonises their allegedly 'anti-social' behaviour. But the UK is not alone in taking this stand: youth policy in most countries is imbued with paradox and contradiction.

Is 'voice' enough?

Many practitioners may claim that the goal of their participative work is to strengthen the 'voice' of young people, to enable them to 'have a say' in what are often adult-dominated situations. In practice, this is actualised where youth workers set up systems or structures to provide a channel for young people's views to be heard. Examples might include school councils, youth forums and youth management committees. Indeed, youth councils have invariably become a 'favoured response' by statutory and voluntary agencies to questions of how to increase youth participation (Matthews 2001). They are certainly popular in schools and are frequently held up as exemplars of meaningful engagement. However, as Matthews (2001: 300) observes:

> Adults often establish youth councils largely because they are perceived to provide tangible opportunities deemed to enable ongoing participation by young people rather than because of demand from young people themselves.

If the models used do not provide structures that 'are sufficiently responsive to provide a sense of control and ownership' (Matthews 2001: 316), there is a danger that they become mere 'talking shops' with limited impact upon the contexts that young people engage with. Fleming and Hudson (2009) argue that such an approach can be interpreted as 'tokenism' that has little value for young people. In this author's own recent research with nearly 100 young people from various schools and youth projects in the East Midlands region (Wood 2009a: 236–238), attempts to promote active citizenship by some schools and participation projects presented a number of interrelated problems. Some of the key issues are listed below:

- Some attempts to engage young people in consultation failed to provide adequate follow up or evidence of acting upon the views gained. This resulted in young people experiencing 'consultation lethargy' – literally a feeling of always being asked for opinions and views with no obvious benefit for young people.
- There was some evidence of failure by youth workers and teachers to introduce a sense of 'realism' to the consultative and participative processes, suggesting that young people could 'change what they wanted' whereas the institutional structures were outside of their control.
- What activities were deemed as 'acceptable acts' of participation were to some extent determined by teachers, youth workers and other message givers. For example, groups of young people could only effectively represent the views of other young people if such views were 'endorsed' by adults in authority.
- For young people, there was a clear sense that power relationships did not change to any meaningful degree. While certain conditions would change in school settings, young people still experienced high levels of disrespect between teachers and students.

There is an overall point to make when considering these difficulties and that is whether we think that promoting a young person's 'voice' is really enough in terms of strengthening participation. In the examples above, the institutions and practitioners promoting active citizenship did so with a commitment to young people. There was no evidence to suggest that they did not seek to improve participation in a meaningful way, but the emphasis on voice ignores the reality of the context of young people's engagement. Schools, for example, are by tradition 'anti-democratic' institutions and pose problems for any attempts to engage in rights-based education (Alderson 1999). They represent, at a micro and local level, the very real power imbalances that face young decision-makers in almost every aspect of their lives. In increasingly target-driven youth work environments, similar difficulties may present themselves.

Thus, while there is ample evidence to suggest that children and young people's participation is being promoted by policy-makers and practitioners, this all still occurs within an overriding message that prioritises an adult view of young people's lives (Hine 2009). Promoting young people's 'voice' depends on more than just establishing structures and systems to enable young people to speak. It also requires practitioners to consider how to make sure that voices are not only *heard* but are *acted upon*. Situating young people's participation in the context of the 'right to participate' may provide a stronger force for promoting participation. The opportunities and capacity of young people to be consulted about and to shape public institutions are often framed as rights and these stem from Article 12 of the UN Convention, as discussed earlier.

The concept of human rights offers a powerful framework for strengthening active citizenship, not least because it is a momentum concept (Hoffman 1997) but also an international legal guarantee. Indeed, Lundy (2007: 940) argues that the case for the increased involvement of young people in decision-making is most compelling when framed within a human rights perspective, suggesting that Article 12 of the UN Convention:

> Can make a unique and powerful contribution to the creation of a children's rights culture . . . one way of sustaining the existing momentum [of involvement] might be to reframe the discourse to reflect the fact that pupil involvement in decision making is a permanent, non-negotiable human right.

If contexts persist which suggest that young people's voices may not really matter, then practitioners can work more effectively with young people to challenge this when they situate their efforts in such a framework.

Conclusion

One of the key values of youth work is to encourage young people's active participation with the aim of supporting them to 'act politically'. This is often realised through citizenship education and programmes of active involvement designed to create opportunities where young people can have a 'voice'. However, key questions become apparent for practitioners engaged in such work. First, this chapter examined the question of 'purpose'. Central to youth work must be an interrogation of *why* we work with young people and to what end. If citizenship education is truly designed to promote the activism and political engagement of young people, this may result in competing and difficult tensions with policy definitions of our work. In response, practitioners may find themselves working to one agenda at the expense of another. Second, this chapter considered the limitations of promoting 'voice' when systems or structures may not be open to listening to young people. However, locating active citizenship education in the context of human rights may provide practitioners with a more robust framework for promoting young people's right to influence and shape the institutions and contexts that impact upon their lives.

In a climate where dominant policy ideas about young people can be defined as contradictory at best, practitioners need to engage in such critical questions in order to strengthen their own ethical commitment to young people's active involvement.

Questions for reflection and discussion

1 Reflect on any efforts to promote active citizenship that you have come across. What evidence is there to suggest that young people's voices are not only heard, but are listened to and acted upon?

2 Consider Case Study 12.1 – the community centre campaign. Can you think of situations where youth workers might face competing tensions in terms of supporting young people to take action? How might practitioners respond?

3 This chapter identifies a tension in the aims of citizenship education between promoting the role of young people as activists and strengthening their social and moral responsibility. Why are these two aims potentially in conflict? Consider how different groups of people (e.g. young people, youth workers, politicians) might value aspects of activism or social and moral responsibility in different ways.

Recommended reading

Dwyer, P. (2004) *Understanding Social Citizenship: Themes and Perspectives*, Bristol: The Policy Press. Provides a useful and accessible introduction to the relationship between citizenship, social policy and social rights. Explores the different traditions of citizenship and provides useful summaries of key ideas.

Heater, D. (2004) *Citizenship: The Civic Ideal in World History, Politics and Education* (3rd edn), Manchester: Manchester University Press. An extensive volume that explores the origins, development and contemporary place of citizenship in a global context.

Wood, J. (2009) 'Education for effective citizenship', in J. Wood and J. Hine (eds) *Work with Young People: Theory and Policy for Practice*, London: Sage. Explores the UK policy context of citizenship education and offers guidance for developing effective citizenship education.

References

Advisory Group on Citizenship (1998) *Education for Citizenship and the Teaching of Democracy in Schools (The Crick Report)*, London: Qualifications and Curriculum Authority.

Alderson, P. (1999) 'Human rights and democracy in schools', *International Journal of Children's Rights*, 7: 185–205.

Andrews, R., Cowell, R. and Downe, J. (2008) 'Support for active citizenship and public service performance: an empirical analysis of English local authorities', *Policy and Politics*, 36: 225–243.

Annette, J. (2008) 'Community involvement, civic engagement and service learning', in J. Arthur, I. Davies and C. Hahn (eds) *The Sage Handbook of Education for Citizenship and Democracy*, London: Sage.

Ballington, J. (2002) 'Voter turnout', in R.L. Pintor and M. Gratschew (eds) *Voter Turnout Since 1945: A Global Report*, Stockholm: IDEA.

BBC (2003a) 'Pupils walk out over war', http://news.bbc.co.uk/1/hi/education/2821 871.stm (accessed 12 March 2003)

BBC (2003b) 'Pupils suspended over protest', http://news.bbc.co.uk/1/hi/england/ 2822533.stm (accessed 12 March 2003)

Brooks, L. (2003) 'Kid power', *Guardian (Weekend Magazine)*, 26 April: 40–44.

Children and Young People's Unit (2001) *Learning to Listen: Core Principles for the Involvement of Children and Young People*, London, Department for Education and Science.

Coffey, A. (2004) *Reconceptualising Social Policy*, Buckingham: Open University Press.

Coleman, S. (2006) *How the Other Half Votes: Big Brother Viewers and the 2005 General Election*, London: Hansard Society.

Crick, B. (2000) *Essays on Citizenship*, London: Continuum.

Cunningham, S. and Lavalette, M. (2004) ' "Active citizens" or "irresponsible truants"? School student strikes against the war', *Critical Social Policy*, 24: 255–269.

Davies, L. (2001) 'Citizenship, education and contradiction', *British Journal of Sociology of Education*, 22: 300–308.

Fleming, J. and Hudson, N. (2009) 'Young people and research: participation in practice', in J. Wood and J. Hine (eds) *Work with Young People: Theory and Policy for Practice*, London: Sage.

France, A. (2007) *Understanding Youth in Late Modernity*, Maidenhead: Open University Press.

Furlong, A. and Cartmel, F. (2007) *Young People and Social Change: New Perspectives* (2nd edn), London: Sage.

Heater, D. (2004) *Citizenship: The Civic Ideal in World History, Politics and Education* (3rd edn), Manchester: Manchester University Press.

Hine, J. (2009) 'Young people's lives: taking a different view', in J. Wood and J. Hine (eds) *Work with Young People: Theory and Policy for Practice*, London: Sage.

Hoffman, J. (1997) 'Citizenship and the state', paper presented at *Citizenship for the 21st Century*, October, University of Central Lancashire, Preston.

Huskins, J. (2003) *Youth Work Support for Schools*, Bristol: John Huskins.

International Institute for Democracy and Electoral Assistance (1999) *Youth Voter Participation: Involving Today's Young in Tomorrow's Democracy*, Stockholm: IIDEA.

Jeffs, T. (2005) 'Citizenship, youth work and democratic renewal', *Encyclopaedia of Informal Education*, www.infed.org/association/citizenship_youth_work_demo cratic_renewal (accessed 1 May 2009).

Lifelong Learning UK (2008) *National Occupational Standards for Youth Work*, www.lluk.org/national-occupational-standards.htm (accessed 12 April 2009).

Lister, R. (2003) *Citizenship: Feminist Perspectives*, 2nd edn, Basingstoke: Palgrave Macmillan.

Lundy, L. (2007) "'Voice' is not enough: conceptualising Article 12 of the United Nations Convention on the Rights of the Child', *British Educational Research Journal*, 33: 927–942.

Marshall, T.H. (1950) *Citizenship and Social Class*, New York: Cambridge University.

Matthews, H. (2001) 'Citizenship, youth councils and young people's participation', *Journal of Youth Studies*, 4: 299–318.

Mulgan, G. and Wilkinson, H. (1997) 'Freedom's children and the rise of generational politics', in G. Mulgan (ed.) *Life After Politics*, London: Fontana.

Pirie, M. and Worcester, R.M. (2000) *The Big Turn-off: Attitudes of Young People to Government, Citizenship and Community*, London: Adam Smith Institute.

Roberts, J. (2009) *Youth Work Ethics*, Exeter: Learning Matters.

Roker, D., Player, K. and Coleman, J. (1999) 'Young people's voluntary and campaigning activities as a source of political education', *Oxford Review of Education*, 25: 185–198.

Rowe, D. (1999) *Youth Work and the Promotion of Citizenship*, London: Citizenship Foundation.

Simpkin, B. (2004) *Participation and Beyond: A Collaborative Research Project Investigating Examples of Participative and Empowering Youth Work*, unpublished Ph.D. thesis, Leicester: De Montfort University.

Turner, B.S. (1993) 'Contemporary problems in the theory of citizenship', in B.S. Turner (ed.) *Citizenship and Social Theory*, London: Sage.

Tyler, M. (2009) 'Managing the tensions', in J. Wood and J. Hine (eds) *Work with Young People: Theory and Policy for Practice*, London: Sage.

UNICEF (2008) *Convention on the Rights of the Child*, www.unicef.org/crc/index_30177.html (accessed 12 December 2008).

Upson, A. (2006) *Perceptions and Experiences of Anti-social Behaviour: Findings from the 2004/05 British Crime Survey*, London: Home Office.

Wallace, C. (2003) 'Introduction: Youth and politics', *Journal of Youth Studies*, 6: 243–245.

Weller, S. (2007) *Teenagers' Citizenship: Experiences and Education*, London: Routledge.

Wilkinson, H. and Mulgan, G. (1995) *Freedom's Children: Work, Relationships and Politics for 18–34 Year Olds in Britain Today*, London: Demos.

Williamson, H. (2009) 'European youth policy and the place of the UK', in J. Wood and J. Hine (eds) *Work with Young People: Theory and Policy for Practice*, London: Sage.

Wood, J. (2009a) *Young People and Active Citizenship: An Investigation*, unpublished Ph.D. thesis, Leicester: De Montfort University.

Wood, J. (2009b) 'Education for effective citizenship', in J. Wood and J. Hine (eds) *Work with Young People: Theory and Policy for Practice*, London: Sage.

Wring, D., Henn, M. and Weinstein, M. (1998) 'Young people and contemporary politics: committed scepticism or engaged cynicism?', *British Elections and Parties Review*, 9: 200–216.

Yates, J. (2009) 'Youth justice: moving in an anti-social direction', in J. Wood and J. Hine (eds) *Work with Young People: Theory and Policy for Practice*, London: Sage.

Young, K. (1999) *The Art of Youth Work*, Lyme Regis: Russell House.

Index

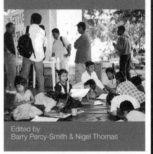

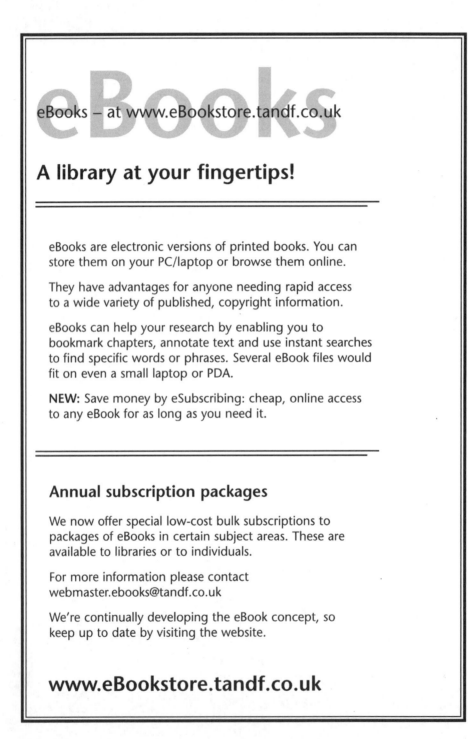